COMPLEMENT

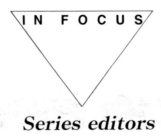

Series editors

David Male
Institute of Psychiatry, De Crespigny Park, Denmark Hill,
London SE5 8AF, UK

David Rickwood
Department of Biology, University of Essex, Wivenhoe Park,
Colchester, Essex CO4 3SQ, UK

Titles published in the series:

*Complement

Enzyme Kinetics

Gene Structure and Transcription

*Immune Recognition

*Lymphokines

*Published in association with the British Society for Immunology.

COMPLEMENT

S.K.A.Law and K.B.M.Reid

MRC Immunochemistry Unit, Department of Biochemistry,
University of Oxford, South Parks Road, Oxford OX1 3QU, UK

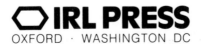
OXFORD · WASHINGTON DC

Published by:
IRL Press Limited
PO Box 1,
Eynsham,
Oxford OX8 1JJ,
UK

1604516

British Library Cataloguing in Publication Data

Law, S.K.A.
   Complement.
   1. Man. Plasma. Complement
   I. Title   II. Reid, K.B.M.   III. Series
   616.07'9

ISBN 1-85221-061-3

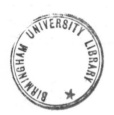

Typeset by Infotype and printed by Information Printing Ltd, Oxford, England.

Preface

Complement is a group of proteins that form the principal effector arm of the humoral immune system. It was initially recognized, at the end of the last century, as the heat-labile factor in serum required along with heat-stable antibody, for bactericidal activity. Today, more than 30 proteins, both in serum and on cell surfaces, have been shown to be closely involved with the complement system. By specific activation steps triggered by the presence of foreign entities, via either the classical or alternative pathways, the complement proteins mediate a set of activities ranging from the initiation of inflammation, neutralization of pathogens, clearance of immune complexes and disruption of cell membranes.

In the past few years, introduction of recombinant DNA technology has allowed more information to be gained concerning the complement proteins with special emphasis on their primary structure. It is now possible to assign the complement components, control proteins and receptors to various superfamilies of structurally related molecules and thus make some correlation between their structures and functions. In addition the gene structures as well as their location in the human genome have been determined for many of the complement proteins. In this book we present a brief introduction to the complement system, covering the basic biochemistry and activation pathways, discuss the different families of proteins in the system and how they interact with each other to mediate the various functions in host defence.

S.K.A.Law
K.B.M.Reid

Acknowledgement

We thank Carolyn Brooks for typing the manuscript rapidly and accurately and for being so patient in view of the many changes and corrections introduced at various stages.

Contents

3. Groups and families of proteins within the complement system

4. Role of complement in health and disease

Abbreviations

C	complement component
C1-Inh	C1-inhibitor
CR	complement receptor
CVF	cobra venom factor
DAF	decay accelerating factor
EBV	Epstein – Barr virus
EGF	epidermal cell growth factor
HANE	hereditary angioneurotic edema
Ig	immunoglobulin
LDL	low density lipoprotein
LFA-1	lymphocyte functional antigen type 1
LHR	long homologous repeat
α_2M	α_2-macroglobulin
MAC	membrane attack complex
MCP	membrane cofactor protein
MHC	major histocompatibility complex
NeF	nephritic factor
NK	natural killer
P	properdin
RCA	regulators of complement activation
RFLP	restriction fragment length polymorphism
SCR	short consensus repeat
SLE	systemic lupus erythematosus

1

Complement

1. Introduction

Complement is a major defence and clearance system in the bloodstream which can be activated via immunoglobulins once a foreign particle or organism has been recognized by antibody. Direct activation of the system can also take place if the particle provides a suitable site for the amplified self-activation of the early acting components. Complement was first described in the 1890s as being principally a heat-labile bactericidal activity in serum which was triggered after the heat-stable antibodies had recognized and bound to the invading micro-organisms. By the 1920s evidence was available showing that the heat-labile bactericidal activity required the presence of at least four serum fractions but, due to the lack of rigorous protein purification methods, little advance was made in the chemical characterization of the numerous components of the system until the early 1960s. Once techniques such as ion-exchange chromatography were readily available it became clear [principally as a result of the work carried out in the laboratories of R.A.Nelson (1) and H.J.Müller-Eberhard (2)] that the immunologically triggered pathway of complement activation (the classical pathway) is composed of eleven distinct plasma proteins. A second activation pathway (the alternative pathway), not necessarily involving antibody, had been proposed by Pillemar in the late 1950s (3,4), but it was not until almost 1970 that evidence of the existence of this pathway was finally accepted (5). Detailed structural, functional and biosynthetic studies on the various components and control proteins regulating the pathways were carried out in the 1970s. This paved the way for the molecular cloning at the cDNA level of all the components, control proteins and many of the receptors associated with the pathways in the period 1982–1987. Thus, in view of the large amount of new information regarding the structure, function, biosynthesis and genetics generated in this relatively short period, it seems appropriate to provide a short but hopefully comprehensive general introduction to the system.

Table 1.1. Plasma proteins involved in the activation of the complement system

	Mol. wt (kd)	Number of chains in plasma form prior to activation	Mol. wt of individual chains (kd)	Chromosome location of gene	Plasma concentration μg/ml	Plasma concentration μM	Enzymatic site in activated form (+) (and natural substrate split)
Classical pathway							
C1q	462	18 (six A + six B + six C)	A: 26.5 B: 26.5 C: 24	1	80	0.17	–
C1r[a]	83	1		1	50	0.30	+ (C1r, C1s)
C1s[a]	83	1		n.k.	50	0.30	+ (C4, C2)
C4	205	3 $(\alpha + \beta + \gamma)$[b]	α: 97 β: 75 γ: 33	12	600	3.00	–
C2	102	1		12	20	0.20	+ (C3, C5)
C3	185	2 $(\alpha + \beta)$[b]	α: 110 β: 75	6	1300	7.02	–
Alternative pathway							
Factor D	24	1		n.k.	1	0.04	+ (B)
Factor B	92	1		6	210	2.20	+ (C3, C5)
C3	185	2 $(\alpha + \beta)$[b]		19	1300	7.02	–
Terminal components							
C5	190	2 $(\alpha + \beta)$[b]	α: 115 β: 75	n.k.	70	0.37	–
C6	120	1		n.k.	64	0.53	–
C7	110	1		n.k.	56	0.51	–
C8	150	3 $(\alpha + \beta + \gamma)$	α: 64 β: 64 γ: 22	1	55	0.36	–
C9	71	1		n.k.	59	0.83	–

n.k. = not known.

[a]C1r and C1s are present in plasma either as a complex with C1q in the composition C1q-C1r$_2$-C1s$_2$ or in the absence of C1q as a C1s-C1r-C1r-C1s tetramer (see text and *Figure 2.2*).

[b]These chains are initially synthesized as a single chain precursor molecule.

1.1 Nomenclature

All proteins associated with the complement system are listed in *Tables 1.1 – 1.3*. The plasma proteins of the classical pathway and terminal attack complex are defined as 'components' and each is given a number and prefaced by 'C'. Thus, C1 – C9 are the components of the classical pathway and terminal membrane attack complex. The membrane attack complex (MAC) is composed of activated C5 along with components C6 – C9. All these components are distinct plasma glycoproteins with the exception of C1, which is a complex of three glycoproteins, the subcomponents of C1: C1q, C1r and C1s. Where there is more than one poly-peptide chain within an unactivated component they are designated α, β and γ. (An exception is the C1q molecule for which the designation A, B and C has been given for the three types of polypeptide chain found in the molecule.) Two of the proteins of the alternative pathway are designated as 'factors' and each is given a letter (factor B and factor D). A third protein of the alternative pathway is properdin. Acceptable abbreviations for these alternative pathway proteins are B, D and P. Two of the control proteins are also designated as 'factors' (factor I and factor H), while the other control proteins are usually referred to by abbreviations of their trivial names, for example C1-Inh for C1-inhibitor.

There are six enzymes, of the serine protease type, associated with the activation and control of the pathways (*Tables 1.1* and *1.2*). Activation steps involving these enzymes are always achieved by very specific limited proteolysis, with only one bond being split at any one step. Control of the activated components is also achieved by splitting of only a limited number of bonds. The enzymatically active forms of components generally have a bar over the symbol, for example $\overline{C1r}$, $\overline{C1s}$. A complex containing an active site may also be written with a bar over the whole complex, for example, $\overline{C1}$ and $\overline{C3b,Bb}$. Fragments generated by limited proteolysis are indicated by suffixed lower case letters, for example C4a and C4b for the activation fragments of C4, C4c and C4d for the degradation fragments of C4b. The receptors are also usually given as abbreviations of their trivial names, for example complement receptor type 1 (the C4b/C3b receptor) is given as CR1.

It should be noted that C4 is activated prior to C2 and C3 and this is merely a reflection of the original numbering given to the fractions containing these components before the order of activation was clearly identified.

1.2 General outline of the complement system

Complement can be activated by two distinct routes, the *classical* and *alternative* pathways (*Figure 1.1*). The component C3 is a major plasma glycoprotein (present at a concentration of 1.3 mg/ml) and it plays a central role in the system being common to both pathways. C3 along with the other 12 plasma glycoproteins shown in *Figure 1.1* and *Table 1.1* constitute the 13 components of the pathways. Components C5 – C9 are designated the terminal components which form the MAC, which is common to both pathways and which is responsible for target cell damage and lysis. Other biologically important functions mediated by the complement system include: (i) the low molecular weight fragments (~ 9000 mol.

Table 1.2. Plasma proteins involved in control of the complement system

Protein	Mol. wt (kd)	Approximate plasma concentration		Specificity	Chromosome location of gene	Role
		μg/ml	μM			
C1-Inh	110	200	1.82	$\overline{C1}r$, $\overline{C1}s$	11	Forms covalent 1:1 complex with both $\overline{C1}r$ and $\overline{C1}s$ and removes them from $\overline{C1}$ complex.
C4 binding protein (C4bp)[a]	500	250	0.45	C4b	1	Accelerates decay of $\overline{C4b2a}$ and acts as cofactor in the cleavage of C4b by factor I.
Factor H	150	480	3.20	C3b	1	Accelerates decay of $\overline{C3bBb}$ and acts as cofactor in the cleavage of C3b by factor I.
Factor I	88	35	0.39	C4b, C3b	4	Protease which inactivates C4b and C3b with the aid of cofactors C4bp, H, CR1 and MCP.
Anaphylatoxin inactivator[b]	310	35	0.11	C3a, C4a, C5a	n.k.	Carboxypeptidase which inactivates the anaphylatoxins C3a, C4a and C5a by removal of a C-terminal arginine residue in each.
S-protein (vitronectin)	83	505	6.08	C5b-9	n.k.	Up to three molecules of S-protein bind to C5b-7 preventing the complex from binding to cell surfaces.
Properdin[c]	220	20	0.09	C3bBb	X	Positive regulator of the alternative pathway which stabilizes the C3/C5 convertases.

n.k. = not known.

MCP = membrane cofactor protein.

[a] C4 binding protein is a disulphide-bonded heptamer of identical subunits of ~70 kd.

[b] Anaphylatoxin inhibitor contains three different polypeptides of mol. wts 83, 55 and 49 kd. The stoichiometric composition of these polypeptides in the protein is not clear.

[c] Properdin is a multimer of a 56 kd subunit; the predominant form contains three or four subunits.

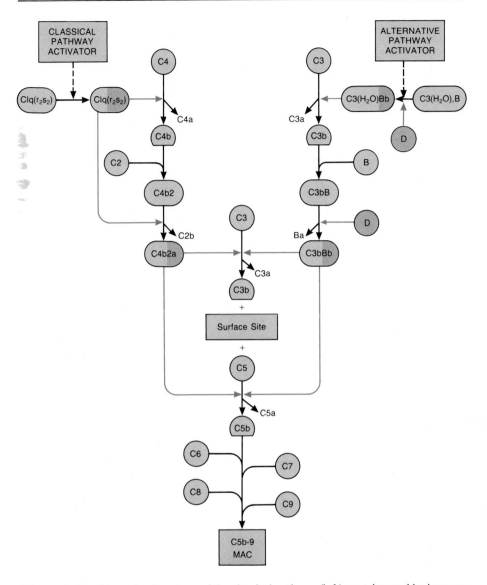

Figure 1.1.   The activation steps of the classical pathway (left) are triggered by immune complexes, while the alternative pathway (right) is activated by a wide variety of compounds and cell surfaces. Enzymatic cleavage is indicated as solid orange lines, and the enzymatically active components are shaded orange.

wt) such as the anaphylatoxins C3a, C4a and C5a, which promote smooth muscle contraction and increase vascular permeability; (ii) the large C4b and C3b fragments, which are involved in binding to the complement activator and can thereafter interact with specific receptors to allow efficient clearance of the activating cell or particle; and (iii) degradation fragments of C3b (iC3b, C3dg,

Table 1.3. Membrane-associated molecules which act as receptors/regulators for fragments[a] of activated complement components

Membrane molecule	Mol. wt[b] (kd)	Fragment specificity	Chromosome location of gene	Principal roles	Major human cell types positive
Complement receptor type 1 (CR1) (four structural allotypes)	type D 250, type B 220, type A 190, type C 160	C3b, C4b	1	Regulation of C3b breakdown, binding of immune complexes to erythrocytes, phagocytosis and accelerates decay of C3/C5 convertases	E, B, G, M
Complement receptor type 2 (CR2)	145	C3d, C3dg, iC3b	1	Regulation of B cell functions, Epstein–Barr virus receptor.	B
Membrane cofactor protein (MCP)	45–70	C3b, C4b	n.k.	Regulation of C3b breakdown.	B, T, N, M
Decay accelerating factor (DAF)	70	C4b2a, C3bBb	1	Accelerates decay of C3/C5 convertases.	E, L, P
Complement receptor type 3 (CR3)	165 (α) 95 (β)	iC3b	n.k. 21	Phagocytosis.	G, M, ϕ
Glycoprotein (p150,95)	150 (α) 95 (β)	iC3b	n.k. 21	Monocyte migration	G, M, ϕ
C3a/C4a receptor	n.k.	C3a, C4a	n.k.	Binding of anaphylatoxins C3a and C4a	G, A
C5a receptor	~45	C5a, C5a-des arg	n.k.	Binding of anaphylatoxin C5a.	G, A, M, ϕ, P
Homologous restriction factor	65	C8, C9	n.k.	Prevention of formation of MAC on homologous cells.	E
C1q receptor	~65	C1q (collagen region)	n.k.	Mediates binding of immune complexes to phagocytic cells. Inhibition of IL-1 expression by B lymphocytes.	B, M, ϕ, P, D

n.k. = not known.
Human cell types: E, erythrocytes; B, B lymphocytes; T, T lymphocytes; M, monocytes; ϕ, macrophages; G, granulocytes; N, neutrophils; L, leukocytes; P, platelets; A, mast cells; D, endothelial cells.
[a]Receptors for intact factor H and Ba have been found on monocytes, B lymphocytes and neutrophils.
[b]All appear to be single chain molecules except CR3 and p150,95 which have non-covalently linked α and β chains.

C3d), which are also important in receptor binding and clearance mechanisms. Other functions include virus neutralization and a possible role in the immune response.

Control of the activated components is mediated partly via the seven control proteins present in plasma (*Table 1.2*) and partly by a variety of membrane bound control proteins and receptors (*Table 1.3*). These membrane proteins bind activated components or fragments of activated components generated by further limited proteolysis. Since many of the activation and control steps involve specific limited proteolysis, it is useful to clearly identify which of the components and control proteins are enzymes. Activation of pro-enzymes C1r, C1s (of the C1 complex) and C2 leads to the formation of enzyme complexes which split C3 and C5. Factors B and D of the alternative pathway are also synthesized as pro-enzymes, although factor D appears to circulate in the blood primarily in its activated form. When factor B is complexed to C3b or C3(H$_2$O) (see Chapter 2, Section 3), it can be split and activated by factor D to eventually yield the enzyme complexes of the alternative pathway which act on C3 and C5 in exactly the same manner as those generated by the classical pathway. After splitting of C5 no other proteolytic events are considered to take place and the lytic C5b-9 complex (MAC) is generated by a self-assembly mechanism.

2. Further reading

Müller-Eberhard,H.J. and Meischer,P.A. (eds) (1985) *Complement*. Springer-Verlag, Berlin.

Reid,K.B.M. and Porter,R.R. (1981) The proteolytic activation systems of complement. *Annu. Rev. Biochem.*, **50**, 433.

Ross,G.D. (ed.) (1986) *Immunobiology of the Complement System: An Introduction for Research and Clinical Medicine*. Academic Press, New York.

Whaley,K. (ed.) (1987) *Complement in Health and Disease*. MTP Press, Lancaster.

2.1 Methods

Harrison,R.A. and Lachman,P.J. (1986) In Wier,D.M., Herzenberg,L.A., Blackwell,C. and Herzenberg,L.A. (eds), *Handbook of Experimental Immunology*. Blackwell Scientific Publications, Oxford, p. 39.1.

Whaley,K. (ed.) (1985) *Methods in Complement for Clinical Immunologists*. Churchill Livingstone Longman Group, Edinburgh.

3. References

1. Nelson,D.S. (1963) *Adv. Immunol.*, **3**, 131.
2. Müller-Eberhard,H.J. (1965) *Adv. Immunol.*, **8**, 2.
3. Pillemar,L., Blum,L., Lepow,I.H., Ross,O.A., Todd,E.W. and Wardlaw,A.C. (1954) *Science*, **120**, 279.
4. Pillemar,L. (1955) *Trans. N.Y. Acad. Sci.*, **17**, 526.
5. Lepow,I.H. (1980) *J. Immunol.*, **125**, 471.

2

Activation and control of the complement system

1. Activation of the classical pathway

The classical pathway is considered to be activated *in vivo* primarily by the interaction of the C1q portion of the C1 complex with immune complexes or
aggregates containing IgG or IgM. Activation of C1 can also be achieved by
its direct interaction with a variety of polyanions (such as bacterial lipopolysaccharides, DNA and RNA), certain small polysaccharides, viral membranes,
etc. but the physiological importance of this type of activitation is not clear. The
C1q molecule, which contains no enzymatic activity, is the portion of the C1
complex which is involved in the recognition and binding of immunoglobulin
activators (1). The molecule contains 18 polypeptide chains (six A, six B and
six C), each of the three types of chain containing a region of 81 amino acids
of collagen-like $(-Gly_x-Xaa-Yaa-)_n$ repeating sequence starting close to the
N-terminal end and which is followed by a C-terminal portion of about 136 amino
acids which are non-collagen-like. Triple helical sections are formed between
the collagen-like regions of the three types of chain and globular 'head' regions
are formed between the non-collagen-like regions of the three types of chain.
Thus, one molecule is composed of six triple helices which are aligned in parallel
throughout half their length and then diverge for the remainder of their length
of triple helical structure to form the connecting strands each of which extends
into one of the six globular 'head' regions (*Figures 2.1* and *2.2*). The enzymatic
activity of C1 is derived by activation of the two molecules of pro-enzyme C1r
and two molecules of pro-enzyme C1s in the $C1r_2$-$C1s_2$ Ca^{2+}-dependent
complex. The purified $C1r_2$-$C1s_2$ complex has an almost rod-like, elongated
shape when viewed in the electron microscope, both C1r and C1s being composed
of two globular domains connected by an elongated structure (*Figure 2.3*), the
larger of the globular domains being considered to contain the catalytic site in
activated C1r or C1s. A model for the C1 complex in which the $C1r_2$-$C1s_2$
complex adopts a distorted 'figure-of-8' structure with the smaller 'interaction'

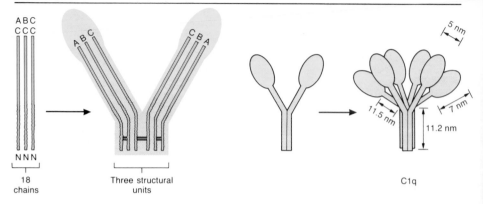

Figure 2.1.   A molecular model of C1q. The molecule consists of 18 chains. The N-terminal portions of the A, B or C chains have collagen-like sequences and adopt a triple helical structure. The C-terminal regions form the globular Fc binding heads. Solid orange bars indicate disulphide bonds.

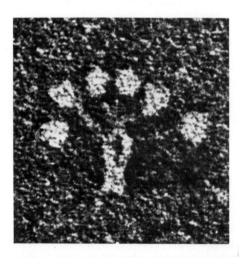

Figure 2.2.   Electron micrograph of a molecule of human C1q showing the apparent separation of proposed structural units (see *Figure 2.1*). This indicates that strong non-covalent bonds holding the units together may be located at the N-terminal ends of the chains. The approximate dimensions of a C1q molecule are indicated in *Figure 2.1*. (The electron microscope picture is from ref. 35.)

domains being located outside the C1q collagen-like strands while the catalytic domains remain closely associated within the collagen-like cage is shown in *Figure 2.3*.

Activation of the C1 complex is under the control of the C1-inhibitor (C1-Inh) (2) which (i) interacts reversibly with the unactivated C1 complex and thus appears to prevent spontaneous activation of pro-enzyme C1r within the complex and (ii) binds covalently with the activated C1r and C1s. The inhibitory effect of C1-Inh can be overcome by efficient activators of the classical pathway such

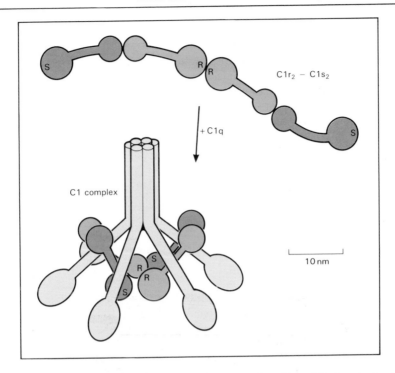

Figure 2.3.   Model of C1r$_2$-C1s$_2$ and the C1 complex. R and S denote the larger catalytic domains of C1r and C1s. It is postulated that the C1 complex is formed by placing the rod-like C1r$_2$-C1s$_2$ across the arms of C1q and bending back around two opposite arms so that both C1s catalytic domains come into contact with the centrally located catalytic domains of C1r (adapted from ref. 36).

as immune complexes. The 'heads' of C1q show a weak binding to the Fc region of monomeric IgG whereas on the presentation of multiple Fc sites of aggregated IgG in immune complexes the strength of the binding of the 'heads' to the multiple Fc regions is dramatically increased. Different IgG isotypes vary in their ability to bind to C1q and activate complement. In man, IgG1 and IgG3 are active, IgG2 is less active and IgG4 inactive. In the case of IgM it is apparently the exposure of binding sites in the Fc regions on interaction with large antigens which allows tight IgM–C1q binding to take place. Thus on the interaction of probably two or more of the 'heads' of C1q with a suitable activator, a conformational change may be induced within the C1 complex releasing it from the inhibitory effect of C1-Inh and allowing auto-activation of pro-enzyme C1r to take place. This is rapidly followed by the activation of pro-enzyme C1s by the C1r due to the close association of the active site of C1r and the activation site of pro-enzyme C1s within the collagen-like 'arms' of C1q (*Figure 2.3*).

The three-chain C4 molecule is then split by C1s at a single point in its α chain to yield the biologically important C4a anaphylatoxin (9000 mol. wt) and the large C4b fragment. The association of C4 with C1 may be via the eight repeating units of 60 amino acids present in the heavy chains of C1r and C1s as outlined in Chapter 3, Section 1. The C4b molecule does not contain an enzymatic site but fulfils at least three important binding functions: (i) the freshly activated C4b has the capacity to bind covalently to hydroxyl or amino groups through a reactive acyl group in its α' chain (see Section 2); (ii) the bound C4b can interact with the CR1 receptor (see Section 6.3) found on a variety of phagocytic cells and could play an important role in immune clearance; and (iii) the C4b can also interact with the N-terminal C2b domain of pro-enzyme C2 in an Mg^{2+}-dependent fashion. If the binding of C2 to C4b occurs close to activated C1s then the C2 is split at one point to yield the non-catalytic C2b (30 000 mol. wt) and the C-terminal catalytic C2a (70 000 mol. wt). The C2b chain is not required for the C3 convertase activity which is mediated via the catalytic site in C2a in the C4b,2a complex.

2. Central role of C3

C3 holds a key position in the complement system since the classical and the alternative pathways merge at the C3 activation step. In the classical pathway, the complex formed by C4b and C2a activates C3 by the proteolytic cleavage of C3 into C3a and C3b (3). C3a is an anaphylatoxin that consists of the first 77 amino acids of the α chain of C3: the remainder of the molecule is C3b. The removal of C3a induces a conformational change in the C3b portion of the molecule which leads to the exposure of an internal thiolester (4), which is buried and quite inaccessible in native C3 (5). The exposed thiolester is extremely reactive and is subjected to nucleophilic attack by water or the hydroxyl or amino groups of other molecules. If the hydroxyl or amino groups belong to molecules of the cell surface, C3b will become covalently bound to the cell by an ester or amide bond (*Figure 2.4*) (6,7).

That C3 has an inert internal thiolester with an ability to form covalently linked complexes with any nucleophile upon activation is a most unusual design in molecular architecture. The ability to bind covalently to any molecule with a hydroxyl or amino group implies that activated C3b can be deposited, potentially, on any biological surface. The ability of C3b to bind to all foreign life forms is clearly a desirable property but its binding to host cells, however, must not take place. This is ensured by the extreme reactive nature of the exposed thiolester. Water, at a concentration of 55 M in the medium, readily hydrolyses the thiolester and puts a limit on the effective range of activated C3b. Thus, C3b activated on the surface of a foreign cell via either the classical or the alternative pathway of complement is restricted to binding to the surface of the same cell or inactivation by water. Host cells, which do not activate the complement pathways, are therefore protected from the binding of C3b.

A similar strategy is employed by C4 and the deposition of C4b on cell surfaces. The reactivity of activated C4b is different from that of C3b in its chemical specificity. The details and significance of this will be discussed in later sections.

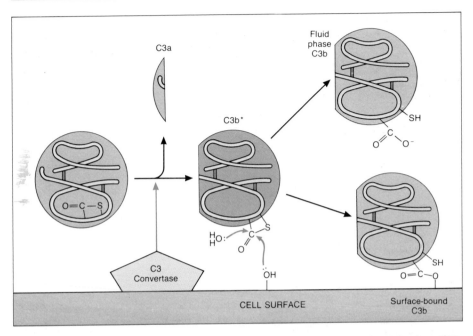

Figure 2.4. Activation of C3. Surface bound C3 convertase splits the α chain of C3 into C3a and C3b. In the process the internal thiolester of the α chain becomes exposed and C3b is regarded as activated (*). The thiolester either reacts with water or with hydroxyl groups on the cell surface, to yield surface bound C3b. C3b* will normally be converted to fluid phase C3b by water before it can diffuse to neighbouring cells. Interchain disulphide bonds are indicated in solid orange.

3. Activation of the alternative pathway

Activation of the alternative pathway does not depend upon antibodies to recognize specific molecules on the target cell surface; rather, it relies on molecular structures on the target cell to upset the very delicate balance of the proteins involved so that their activation and deposition are focused on its surface.

   C3 is continuously activated at a slow rate in the fluid phase. It could be the serum proteases that convert C3 to C3b, or the small nucleophiles, or water, that gain access to the internal thiolester, or simply the perturbation of the C3 structure by any means leading to the exposure of the thiolester (8 – 11) (*Figure 2.5*). C3 with a hydrolysed thiolester without the loss of its C3a fragment is called C3i, also often designated as C3(H$_2$O), which has a molecular conformation like C3b and is able to form a C3 convertase with factor B in the presence of factor D (10). It must be stressed that all these processes only operate at a low level, and the probability that the activated C3b* or C3i* (see *Figure 2.5*) will bind covalently to a cell surface is even lower. However, if a C3b or C3i is deposited on an activating surface of the alternative pathway, it can serve as a seed for the positive amplification loop which operates explosively (12,13). *In vivo*, where

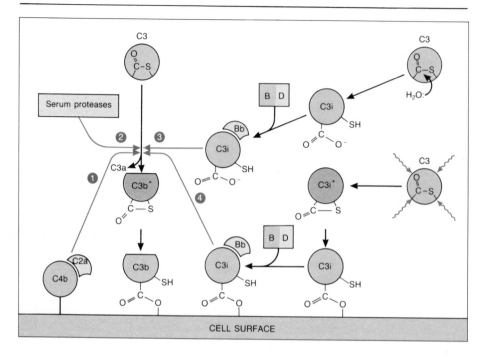

Figure 2.5. The most important mechanism of the initial deposition of C3b on an alternative pathway activator *in vivo* is probably by the C4b2a enzyme of the classical pathway (1). Other mechanisms include: (2) cleavage of C3 by serum proteases, (3) conversion of C3 into C3i by water or other small nucleophiles, and (4) perturbation of C3 leading to direct binding of C3i on the cell surface.

both the classical and alternative pathways of complement act in concert to fight against infections, the most likely mechanism to deposit the initial C3b on a foreign cell surface involves the classical pathway.

It may easily be appreciated that the enzymes, C3b,Bb and C3i,Bb, if left unchecked, would quickly lead to the activation of all C3 and factor B by a positive feedback loop. However, there are control proteins in serum. Factor H operates in two ways to inactivate the C3b,Bb enzyme: (i) it accelerates the dissociation of Bb from C3b (14); and (ii) it serves as a cofactor for factor I, a serine protease, which cleaves C3b into iC3b, which can no longer form the C3 convertase with factor B (15). Hence, in normal circumstances, the activation of C3 is kept at a low level in the fluid phase (*Figure 2.6a*). Indeed, individuals with a deficiency of factor I have a low C3 level, about 10% that of normal, and were first detected as a deficiency for C3.

A minute amount of C3 activated by schemes 2, 3 and 4 as shown in *Figure 2.5* could be deposited on cell surfaces in a random and non-specific fashion. Non-activating surfaces of the alternative pathway permit the control proteins to prevent the formation of the C3b,Bb complex, either by the displacement of Bb from C3b or by the cleavage of C3b into iC3b (*Figure 2.6b*). Activating

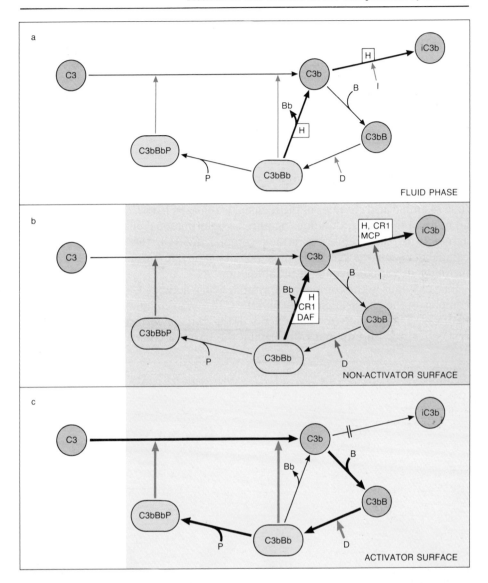

Figure 2.6.   The alternative pathway amplification loop is restricted to certain surfaces by a balance of interactions between complement proteins. **(a)** In the fluid phase activation is curtailed by efficient cleavage of C3b by factor I and cofactors. **(b)** Surface bound C3b on non-activators is regulated similarly and in addition C3bBb is actively dissociated by factor H, CR1 and DAF. **(c)** On activator surfaces these two regulatory pathways are inhibited and rapid deposition of C3b on the surface ensues.

surfaces, however, have the common but undefined property of providing a 'protected site' which retards the action of the control proteins on C3b,Bb, thus allowing the positive feedback C3-activation loop to operate on the surface (*Figure 2.6c*).

Since the initial deposition of C3b or C3i is non-specific, some of the C3b or C3i molecules may become covalently bound to the surface of a host cell. To ensure against the possibility of setting the amplification loop in motion, host cells have three membrane proteins, CR1 (16), decay accelerating factor (DAF) (17) and membrane cofactor protein (MCP) (18), that have functions similar to those of factor H to actively prevent the formation of the C3b,Bb complex.

4. Activation of C5

C5 is a homologue of C3 and C4. It is therefore not surprising that the activation of C5 resembles those of C3 and C4. A small fragment, C5a, consisting of the first 74 amino acid residues of the α chain, is released from C5b. Though lacking an internal thiolester, C5b does acquire a conformational change to initiate the assembly of the membrane attack complex (MAC), the terminal steps of complement activity. C5a is the most potent anaphylatoxin and it is an important mediator in various events in inflammation.

The enzymes in the complement system which activate C5 are the C4b,2a,3b complex of the classical pathway and the C3b,Bb,3b complex of the alternative pathway. The proteolytic components in the two convertases are C2a and Bb respectively, with C4b and C3b playing the parts of cofactors. The assembly

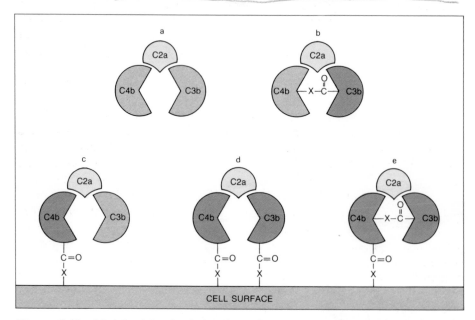

Figure 2.7. Models of the classical pathway C5 convertase. The trimolecular complex may be formed in solution (a,b) or on a cell surface (c–e). There is evidence that the activated thiolester of C3b links to C4b (b and e) and the most recently proposed model is e, which is yet to be proven correct. It is very probable that complexed C3b and C4b differ from their molecular configuration in the free form. "X" could either be an "O" or "NH", depending on the ester or amide nature of the bond.

of these two C5 convertases is complicated since each has three complement protein components, two of which may be required to covalently link to other macromolecules. All the possible arrangements of the components of the classical C5 convertase are shown in *Figure 2.7*. An equivalent set of figures could be drawn for the C5 convertase of the alternative pathway.

In the most recent model (e) C4b is required to be covalently bound to a cell surface macromolecule and C3b to be bound covalently to C4b. If this model is correct, then it is necessary to postulate that there is a specific site on C4b to which C3b binds. A covalent complex between C4b and C3b has been shown to exist and the acceptor site on C4b was shown to be on its α' chains. Whether this complex can interact with C2a to mediate C5 activation is not yet known.

5. Activation of the membrane attack complex (MAC) C5b-9

The lytic activity of complement was the first well-defined function attributed to the system and it is now well established that the five plasma glycoproteins C5 – C9 undergo a hydrophilic – amphiphilic transition to produce the typical cytolytic complement lesion seen in model systems using red blood cells or liposomes as targets (*Figure 2.8*). Together the terminal components can produce a complex of $1-2 \times 10^6$ molecular weight referred to as the MAC. The MAC forms transmembrane channels which displace lipid molecules and other constituents, thus disrupting the phospholipid bilayer of target cells leading to osmotic cell lysis.

The only proteolytic event in the formation of the MAC appears to be the splitting of C5 to C5a plus C5b by the C5 convertases of either pathway (Chapter 1, *Figure 1.1*). The freshly activated C5b, loosely bound to C3b, binds to C6 to form a C5b-6 complex and then to C7 to form a C5b-7 complex which has a transient binding site for membrane surfaces (*Figure 2.9*) and becomes dissociated from C3b. If the C5b-7 complex fails to rapidly bind to a membrane surface via sites in C6 and C7, its potential cytolytic activity is lost and self-aggregation takes place in the fluid phase. The binding of the three-chain C8 molecule (α, 64 000; β, 64 000; γ, 22 000 mol wts, respectively) to C5b-7 takes place via a specific C5b recognition site on C8β. After C8 is bound the C8α chain directs the incorporation of C9 to form C5b. Although the C5b-8 complex is capable of slowly lysing red blood cells as well as certain nucleated cells, its principal role would appear to be to act as a receptor for C9 and behave as a catalyst in C9 polymerization to yield the highly effective C5b-9 cytolytic complex (*Figure 2.10*). The manner by which C5b-8 binding of one molecule of C9 allows a high affinity C9 – C9 interaction is not absolutely clear, but it is likely that the relatively hydrophobic sections of the C-terminal half of C9 become inserted into the phospholipid of the target membrane. The MAC has a composition of C5b-8(C9)$_n$ (where n may lie between 1 and 18) but the type of lesion seen is dependent upon the availability of monomeric C9 (19). In a model system using

a

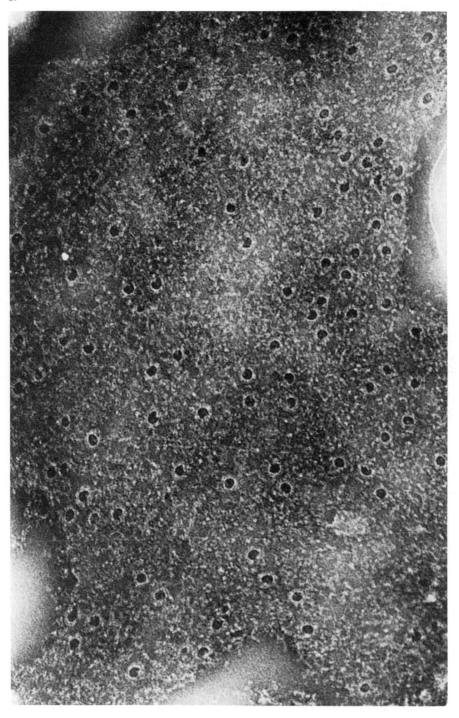

b

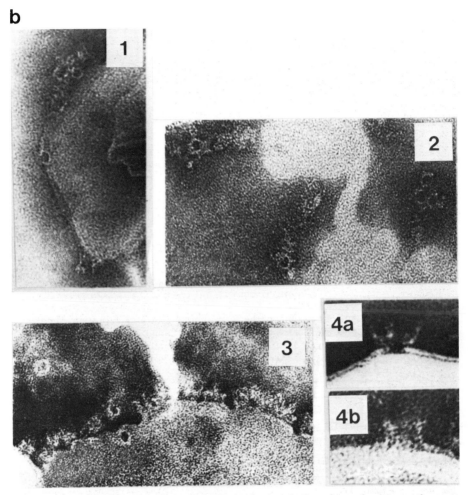

Figure 2.8. (a) Electron micrograph of complement lesions formed on an erythrocyte membrane, treated with rabbit antibody and guinea pig complement. The lesions are stable and uniform but the size (i.d. 8.5 – 11 nm) varies with the species of complement used (electron micrograph kindly supplied by Dr E.A.Munn). **(b)** Electron micrographs of liposomes (artificial membranes) after treatment with complement components (from ref. 37 where full experimental details are given). The electron micrographs show: (1) sphingomyelin – cholesterol liposomes + C$\overline{567}$ + C8 + C9, with the lesions seen in profile; (2) sphingomyelin liposomes + C$\overline{567}$ + C8 + C9, with groups of lesions in top view detached from the liposomes; (3) lecithin liposome + C$\overline{567}$ + C8 + C9 showing lesions in top view, profile and detached; (4) higher magnification views of lesions seen in profile from a lecithin liposome (a) and from a sphingomyelin cholesterol liposome (b).

purified proteins, typical cylinder-like membrane lesions are seen (*Figure 2.8*) at a C9:C5b-8 ratio of 6:1, whereas at a ratio of 1:1 only a network of protein aggregates are seen and no lesions are apparent. However, even at the low C9 input there was efficient cell lysis, indicating that the ring-like lesions may not be a pre-requisite for cell lysis and that complexes with a low number of C9

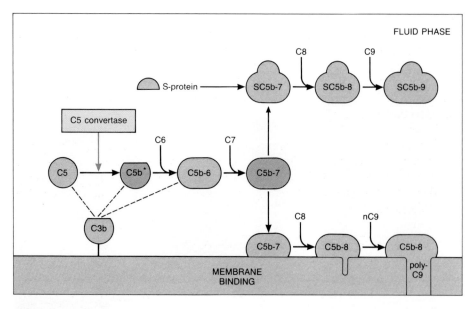

Figure 2.9.   Scheme of assembly of the MAC and its control by S-protein. Metastable forms of C5b and C5b-7 are shaded tan. C5b is loosely bound to membrane C3b. Initial attachment of the assembling MAC is via a transient binding site in C5b-7.

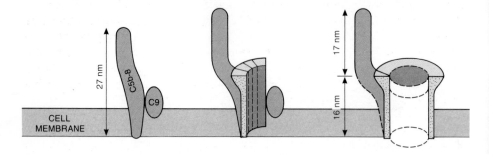

Figure 2.10.   A model of the MAC, in which C5b-8 directs polymerization of poly C9 channels which traverse the cell membrane (adapted from ref. 32).

molecules may simply produce smaller, but effective, hydrophobic membrane channels (20,21).

6. Control of the complement system

As with any cascade system which can deliver a rapid and amplified response via the initial activation at a relatively small number of sites, the complement system requires fine control at several levels. An indication of the amplification factors involved comes from the estimate that activation of one C1 complex by antibody at a cell surface can result in the generation of several hundred C3b molecules which can become distributed over a relatively large area of the activating cell. The amplification in this case is due to the feedback of C3b into the alternative pathway which generates more of the C3 convertase $\overline{C3b,Bb}$ (*Figure 2.5*). Thus, it can be seen that levels of the functionally important C3 molecule could be rapidly reduced to zero in the absence of suitable control mechanisms.

The activated components of the pathways come under the control of various regulatory proteins and enzymes as discussed in Sections 6.1–6.5 but, in addition, it should be noted that the C3 and C5 convertases decay quite rapidly and that C4b, C3b and C5b-7 display only transient ability to bind to suitable target surfaces.

6.1 C1-inhibitor (C1-Inh) and the C1 complex

C1-Inh is considered to interact reversibly with the unactivated C1 complex and prevent spontaneous activation of pro-enzyme C1r in the complex. The evidence for this role for C1-Inh stems from the observation that highly purified C1 appears to activate spontaneously but does not do so when in the presence of C1-Inh at concentrations of the inhibitor found in serum. After activation of C1 has taken place, for example by its binding to immune complexes, the C1-Inh rapidly forms a covalent 1:1 complex with both the activated $\overline{C1r}$ and $\overline{C1s}$, probably via the catalytic sites, resulting in the release of a (C1-Inh)-$\overline{C1r}$-$\overline{C1s}$-(C1-Inh) complex (22). This prevents over-activation of the classical pathway and efficiently removes $\overline{C1r}$ and $\overline{C1s}$ from the activator-$\overline{C1}$ complex, thus leaving the collagen-regions of C1q free to interact with the widespread C1q receptor and fulfil a number of effector functions which include cell-mediated cytotoxicity, inhibition of interleukin-1 production, stimulation of oxidative metabolism in polymorpho-nuclear leukocytes and Fc-receptor-mediated phagocytosis.

C1-Inh is a member of the serpin family of inhibitors (23) and, although it inhibits a variety of other activated plasma proteases (including kallikrein, plasmin, Hageman factor and factor XI), it is likely that its major role lies in control of complement activation since it is the only plasma inhibitor directed against $\overline{C1r}$ and $\overline{C1s}$ (22). The importance of $\overline{C1}$-Inh is illustrated from the study of patients suffering from hereditary angioneurotic edema (HANE) (24). In HANE there is a deficiency of $\overline{C1}$-Inh which is inherited as an autosomal dominant trait and is associated with attacks of localized, increased vascular permeability and it is suspected that the kinin-like activity in the disease may emanate from an over activation of C2 and/or bradykinin.

6.2 Anaphylatoxin inactivator

The anaphylatoxins C3a, C4a and C5a are all peptides, 74–77 amino acid residues long, released from the splitting of a single Arg–X bond in the α chains of C3, C4 and C5, respectively upon activation of the complement system. These peptides mediate many inflammatory responses and have also been implicated in the regulation of immune responses (25). A variety of cells possess receptors for the anaphylatoxins and binding to these receptors brings about vascular permeability changes, induction of smooth muscle contraction and release of histamine from mast cells and basophils. The spasmogenic activities of the three anaphylatoxins are in the order C5a > C3a > C4a. These activities are rapidly controlled in the blood by the anaphylatoxin inactivator (serum carboxypeptidase N), which can remove the C-terminal Arg from each of the anaphylatoxins. The C-terminal Arg found in C3a and C4a is essential for activity, but C5a, lacking its C-terminal Arg, still contains considerable chemotactic activity. Thus, C5a is probably the most important of the anaphylatoxins in terms of normal host defence mechanisms.

6.3 Factor I and its cofactors and related regulatory proteins

6.3.1 Factor I

Factor I is a highly specific serine protease which is involved with the regulation of the C3/C5 convertases of either pathway. Using C4b-binding protein (C4bp) or H as a cofactor it splits the α' chains of C4b or C3b, respectively, causing rapid loss of the biological activities associated with C3b and C4b, which includes their roles in the C3/C5 convertases.

The following section is concerned with the proteins which bind to C4b and C3b (the major fragments released on the activation of C4 and C3). Some of these proteins are cofactors for factor I, while the function of others is limited to that of binding to C3 and C4 fragments.

6.3.2 C4b-binding protein (C4bp) and factor H

C4bp is composed of seven identical chains and appears in the electron microscope as a 'spider-like shape' composed of seven thin, elongated, flexible arms linked to a small ring-like core. [This unusual structure is discussed in Chapter 3, Section 4 (26,27).] The C4bp molecule has multiple binding sites for C4b, each of which appear to be located close to the peripheral tip of each arm. By virtue of this binding capacity C4bp can inhibit the formation of the C3 convertase (i.e. C4b,2a), and it can also accelerate decay of the convertase possibly by displacing C2a. When C4bp is bound to C4b it can act as a cofactor for factor I, allowing it to efficiently split the C4b at two positions to yield C4c and C4d.

Factor H is a single-chain glycoprotein and is the most abundant cofactor in blood which binds C3b, thus regulating the many functions associated with C3b. The binding of C3b appears to involve the N-terminal third of the molecule as discussed in Chapter 3, Section 4. The binding of factor H to C3b greatly accelerates the decay of C3b,Bb and C3b,Bb,P, and it is likely that it also regulates the C5 convertase since it competes with the binding of C5 to C3b. In a similar fashion to the C4bp-C4b interaction in the classical pathway, factor H acts as a cofactor in the splitting of C3b (and C3i) by factor I, allowing cleavage

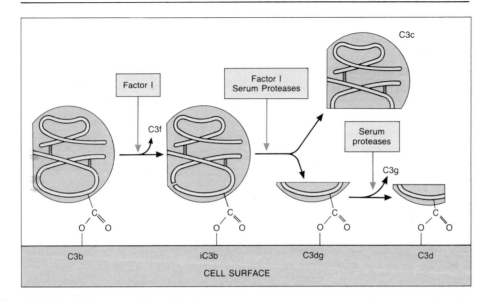

Figure 2.11. Breakdown of C3b. (**1**) Membrane bound C3b with an α chain of 106 kd and a β chain of 75 kd is acted on by factor I and cofactors to release C3f (3 kd), cleaving the α chain into 40 kd and 63 kd fragments. (**2**) Serum proteases or factor I in association with CR1 cleave the α chain again (α_1 23 kd: α_2 40 kd) to release C3c and leave C3dg (40 kd) attached to the membrane. (**3**) Exogenous proteases release C3g (5 kd) to leave C3d (35 kd). Interchain disulphide bonds are indicated in solid orange.

of the α' chain of C3b in two positions to yield iC3b (*Figure 2.11*). The further proteolysis of iC3b to yield the C3c and C3dg fragments is thought to involve factor I as well as other trypsin-like enzymes such as plasmin.

6.3.3 Complement receptor type 1 (CR1), complement receptor type 2 (CR2), membrane cofactor protein (MCP) and decay acceleration factor (DAF)

Control of the C3 convertases are also mediated by four membrane-bound proteins. CR1 and CR2 are true membrane proteins in that they are anchored to the membrane by a hydrophobic transmembrane segment (28). DAF does not have a transmembrane segment but is bound to the membrane by a glycolipid anchor (29,30). Presumably it is synthesized as a membrane protein whose extracellular moiety is then transferred to phosphatidylinositol molecule by a specific reaction. How the MCP is bound to the membrane is not known.

As seen in *Table 1.3*, the four proteins regulate the C3 convertase differently in their ability to mediate either the decay acceleration reaction, or the factor-I-mediated cleavage of C4b or C3b, or both. They do not have the same cellular expression. Perhaps because of their sole activity as regulators of the C3 convertases, and hence as a protective agent of host cells from the incidental activation of the complement pathways, MCP and DAF are found on a wide range of cell types. CR1 is more versatile. Its presence on erythrocyte surfaces has an important role in the clearance of immune complexes. Immune complexes, via their covalently bound C3b and C4b, bind to the CR1 on erythrocytes which serve as a carrier of immune complexes to sites, such as the liver and the spleen, where they are removed from circulation (31). CR1 is also found on phagocytes, where it mediates the binding of opsonized targets to initiate the phagocytic process. CR2 is found predominantly on B lymphocytes. Its interaction with C3dg may be important in regulating B cell function. Details of the functional activity are not well understood.

6.4 Homologous restriction factor and S-protein (vitronectin) in control of the membrane attack complex

Certain activators of complement, such as immune complexes, do not contain lipid bilayers to which C5b-7 can bind and other activators, such as yeast cell walls or complement-resistant bacteria, appear to be shielded in some manner from the transient membrane binding activity of C5b-7. The C5b-7 complex present in the fluid phase can in certain cases bind to 'bystander' host cells which can then be lysed by the action of C8 and C9. To avoid this situation, control of the C5b-7 complex is mediated by several plasma inhibitors (such as lipo-proteins, antithrombin III and the S-protein) and a membrane-bound inhibitor which binds homologously to C8 and C9. Of the plasma inhibitors, the S-protein is the most efficient and probably the major controlling factor of the lytic potential of the MAC in plasma (32). The S-protein, a single chain plasma glycoprotein of 80 000 molecular weight has recently been shown to be identical to the 'spreading protein' called vitronectin. Up to three molecules of S-protein can bind to the C5b-7 complex which contains the transient binding site for cell surface lipids. The binding of S-protein thus prevents the complex from binding to cell surfaces and therefore protects bystander cells against lysis by the MAC. The resulting fluid phase SC5b-7 can bind C8 and C9 but extensive polymeriza-tion of C9 does not take place since the final product always appears to have the composition $SC5b-9_3$. The S-protein containing complexes may be cleared from the circulation via S-protein receptors present on a wide variety of cells.

The finding that complement is more efficient in lysing heterologous red blood cells rather than autologous red cells appears to be related to the presence of a C8/C9-binding protein in the membranes of the host cells. This membrane protein, which has been designated homologous restriction factor, has a molecular weight of 65 000 when isolated from solubilized red blood cell membranes and appears to show a limited immunochemical relationship to C8 and C9 (33).

6.5 Stabilizing role of properdin

Properdin was the first of the alternative pathway proteins to be identified and with the result that the alternative pathway was, and sometimes still is, referred to as the 'properdin' pathway. It is present in plasma in the form of a mixture of cyclic polymers of a 56 000 molecular weight chain, with tetramers and trimers being the predominant species (33,34). The monomer appears highly asymmetric

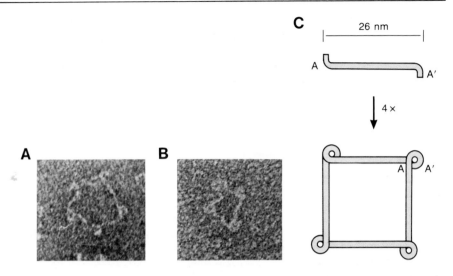

Figure 2.12. Electron micrographs of properdin oligomers: (**A**) cyclic pentamer, (**B**) cyclic tetramer. Magnification is ×320 000, the dimension of a monomer was estimated from measurements made on 136 sides of 34 tetramers, giving values of 24 ± 2 nm as the mean length and 2.5 ± 3 nm as the mean width (at all points except the ends). (**C**) A model for a cyclic tetramer is shown where complementary binding sites (A and A′) are localized at ends of the monomeric properdin 26 nm in length and 3 nm in width. (From ref. 38.)

when viewed in the electron microscope (26 nm × 3 nm) and it associates in a head-to-tail fashion to form the polymers (*Figure 2.12*). Properdin is, to date, the only control protein in normal plasma which displays a stabilizing rather than a disruptive or degradative role. It does this by binding to C3b in the C3b,Bb complex thus significantly increasing the life of the C3/C5 convertases.

7. Further reading

7.1 C1 activation

Arlaud,G.J., Colomb,M.G. and Gagnon,J. (1987) *Immunol. Today*, **8**, 106.
Schumaker,V.N., Zavodsky,P. and Poon,P.H. (1987) *Annu. Rev. Immunol.*, **5**, 21.

7.2 Activation of the complement pathways

Lachmann,P.J. and Hughes-Jones,N.C. (1985) In Müller-Eberhard,H.J. and Meischer,P.A. (eds), *Complement*. Springer-Verlag, Berlin, p. 147.
Pangburn,M.K. (1986) In Ross,G.D. (ed.), *Immunobiology of the Complement System*. Academic Press, New York, p. 45.
Reid,K.B.M. (1986) *Essays Biochem.*, **22**, 27.

7.3 Internal thiolester and covalent binding of C3

Law,S.K.A. (1983) *Annu. N. Y. Acad. Sci.*, **421**, 246.
Tack,B.F. (1985) In Müller-Eberhard,H.J. and Miescher,P.A. (eds), *Complement*. Springer-Verlag, Berlin, p. 49.

7.4 Membrane attack complex

Müller-Eberhard,H.J. (1986) *Annu. Rev. Immunol.*, **4**, 503.
Podack,E.R. (1986) In Ross,G.D. (ed.), *Immunobiology of the Complement System.*
Academic Press, New York, p. 115.

8. References

1. Reid,K.B.M. (1983) *Biochem. Soc. Trans.*, **11**, 1.
2. Ziccardi,R.J. (1985) *J. Immunol.*, **134**, 2559.
3. Müller-Eberhard,H.J., Dalmasso,A.P. and Calcott,M.A. (1966) *J. Exp. Med.*, **124**, 33.
4. Tack,B.F., Harrison,R.A., Janatova,J., Thomas,M.L. and Prahl,J.W. (1980) *Proc. Natl. Acad. Sci. USA*, **77**, 5764.
5. Pangburn,M.K. and Müller-Eberhard,H.J. (1980) *J. Exp. Med.*, **152**, 1102.
6. Law,S.K. and Levine,R.P. (1977) *Proc. Natl. Acad. Sci. USA*, **74**, 2701.
7. Law,S.K., Lichtenberg,N.A. and Levine,R.P. (1979) *J. Immunol.*, **123**, 1388.
8. Nicol,P.A.E. and Lachmann,P.J. (1973) *Immunology*, **24**, 259.
9. Fearon,D.T. and Austen,K.F. (1975) *J. Immunol.*, **115**, 1357.
10. Pangburn,M.K., Schreiber,R.D. and Müller-Eberhard,H.J. (1981) *J. Exp. Med.*, **154**, 856.
11. Law,S.K.A. (1983) *Biochem. J.*, **211**, 381.
12. Fearon,D.T. and Austen,K.F. (1977) *J. Exp. Med.*, **146**, 22.
13. Pangburn,M.K. and Müller-Eberhard,H.J. (1978) *Proc. Natl. Acad. Sci. USA*, **75**, 2416.
14. Whaley,K. and Ruddy,S. (1976) *Science*, **193**, 1101.
15. Pangburn,M.K., Schreiber,R.D. and Müller-Eberhard,H.J. (1977) *J. Exp. Med.*, **146**, 257.
16. Fearon,D.T. (1979) *Proc. Natl. Acad. Sci. USA*, **76**, 5867.
17. Nicholson-Weller,A., Bunge,J., Fearon,D.T., Weller,P.F. and Austen,K.F. (1982) *J. Immunol.*, **129**, 184.
18. Seya,T., Turner,J.R. and Atkinson,J.P. (1986) *J. Exp. Med.*, **163**, 837.
19. Podack,E.R., Tschopp,J. and Müller-Eberhard,H.J. (1982) *J. Exp. Med.*, **156**, 268.
20. Bhakdi,S. and Tranum-Jenson,J. (1986) *J. Immunol.*, **136**, 2999.
21. Dankert,J.R. and Esser,A.F. (1985) *Proc. Natl. Acad. Sci. USA*, **82**, 2128.
22. Sim,R.B. and Reboul,A. (1981) *Methods Enzymol.*, **80C**, 43.
23. Bock,S.C., Skriver,K., Nielsen,E., Thogersen,H.-C., Wiman,B., Donaldson,V.H., Eddy,R.L., Marriana,J., Radziejewski,E., Huber,R., Shows,T.B. and Magnussen,S. (1986) *Biochemistry*, **25**, 4292.
24. Donaldson,V.H., Harrison,R.A., Rosen,F.S., Bing,D.H., Kindness,G., Canar,J., Wagner,C.G. and Awad,S. (1985) *J. Clin. Invest.*, **75**, 124.
25. Hugli,T.E. (1981) *CRC Crit. Rev. Immunol.*, **1**, 321.
26. Dahlback,B., Smith,C.A. and Müller-Eberhard,H.J. (1983) *Proc. Natl. Acad. Sci. USA*, **80**, 3461.
27. Zaccardi,R.J., Dahlback,B. and Müller-Eberhard,H.J. (1984) *J. Biol. Chem.*, **259**, 13674.
28. Klickstein,L.B., Wong,W.W., Smith,J.A., Weis,J.H., Wilson,J.G. and Fearon,D.T. (1987) *J. Exp. Med.*, **165**, 1095.
29. Caras,I.W., Davitz,M.A., Rhee,L., Weddell,G., Martin,D.W.Jr and Nussenzweig,V. (1987) *Nature*, **325**, 545.
30. Medof,M.E., Lublin,D.M., Holers,V.M., Ayers,D.J., Getty,R.R., Leyham,J.F., Atkinson,J.P. and Tykocinski,M.L. (1987) *Proc. Natl. Acad. Sci. USA*, **84**, 2007.
31. Cornakoff,J.B., Hebert,L.A., Smead,W.L., Vanaman,M.E., Birmingham,D.J. and Waxman,F.J. (1983) *J. Clin. Invest.*, **71**, 236.

32. Podack,E.R., Preissner,K.T. and Müller-Eberhard,H.J. (1984) *Acta Pathol. Microbiol. Scand.* Series C (Suppl. 248) **92**, 89.
33. Zalman,L.S., Wood,L.M. and Müller-Eberhard,H.J. (1986) *Proc. Natl. Acad. Sci. USA,* **83**, 6975.
34. Reid,K.B.M. (1981) *Methods Enzymol.,* **80C**, 143.
35. Knobel,H.R., Villiger,W. and Isliker,H. (1975) *Eur. J. Immunol.,* **5**, 78.
36. Arlaud,G.J., Colomb,M.G. and Gagnon,J. (1987) *Immunol. Today,* **8**, 106.
37. Lachmann,P.J., Bowyer,D.E., Nicol,P., Dawson,R.M.C. and Munn,E.A. (1973) *Immunology,* **24**, 135.
38. Smith,C.A., Pangburn,M.K., Vogel,C.W. and Müller-Eberhard,H.J. (1984) *J. Biol. Chem.,* **259**, 4582.

3

Groups and families of proteins within the complement system

1. The serine proteases of the complement system

All enzymes participating in the major steps concerned with activation (C1r, C1s, C2, factor B, factor D) and control (factor I), of the complement pathways belong to the family of mammalian serine proteases which include the digestive enzymes such as chymotrypsin and trypsin. A feature which these enzymes share is the presence of a serine protease 'domain' of approximately 23 000 molecular weight with a characteristic 'triad' of active site residues His-57, Asp-102, Ser-195 (chymotrypsin numbering) comprising the charge relay system, indicating evolution from a common ancestor (1). (An exception in the group of enzymes associated with the complement system is the anaphylatoxin inactivator, carboxypeptidase N, which removes the C-terminal Arg from the anaphylatoxins C3a, C4a and C5a. Also, the processing enzymes which are involved in the conversion of the single chain precursor forms of C3, C4 and C5 to the major plasma forms of two, three and two chain molecules, respectively, are as yet uncharacterized but are likely to involve several intracellular enzymes, some with tryptic-like specificity and at least one with a carboxypeptidase-B-like activity.)

The complement serine proteases are synthesized and usually secreted as pro-enzymes. However, both factor D and factor I appear to circulate in the blood primarily in their activated forms since significant amounts of the pro-enzyme forms have not yet been consistently demonstrated in plasma or serum samples, even after the addition of a wide spectrum of protease inhibitors. As can be seen from the overall structures of most of the activated forms of complement enzymes (and many of those in another cascade system—the blood clotting system), regulatory serine proteases often differ from the broadly specific, digestive serine proteases (such as trypsin) by having a large N-terminal polypeptide chain (as distinct from a small activation peptide) added to the serine protease domain (*Figure 3.1*). In the case of C2 and factor B, 'extra' segments are also found within the serine protease region. These extra segments are clearly involved in the

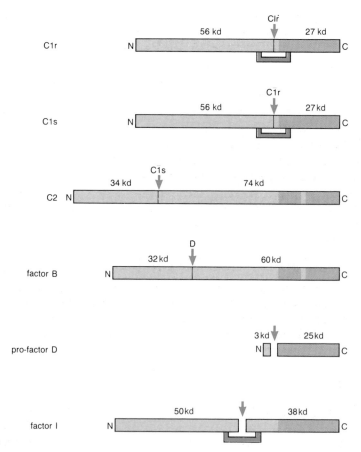

Figure 3.1. The serine proteases involved in activation and control of the complement system. C1r̄ denotes a single chain form of C1r with proteolytic activity. The active site residues (His-57: Asp-102: Ser-195) are encoded in the serine protease domain shaded orange. The gaps in C2 and B represent sequences encoded by an extra exon absent from other members of this family.

recognition and binding to suitable substrates and in control of specificity of the regulatory enzymes. A feature of the complement serine proteases is their high specificity for a particular protein substrate which usually involves one, or at most three (in the case of factor I on C3b), bonds in another complement component. Thus, limited proteolysis of pro-enzymes C1r, C1s, C2 and factor B by C1r̄, C1̄r, C1̄s and factor D, respectively (*Figures 1.1* and *3.1*), under physiological conditions requires the formation of a cation-dependent protein complex of at least two components to provide activation; the enzymes involved in the activation of pro-enzyme forms of factor D and factor I have not yet been characterized.

1.1 C1r and C1s

In the activated forms of C1r and C1s the non-catalytic heavy chain (A chain,

55 000 mol. wt), derived from the N-terminal end of the pro-enzyme, contains a potential growth factor domain and two different pairs of internal repeating sequences. The catalytic chain (B chain, 27 000 mol. wt) contains the active site residues characteristic of the serine protease family (2,3). The first set of repeating sequences (occupying approximately residues 10–80 and 185–255) in both the A chains of C1r and C1s do not appear to show similarity with portions of any other characterized serine proteases and thus, could be involved with the activation and/or control of specificity of the enzymes. The epidermal growth factor (EGF)-like domain found between these repeats is relatively widespread in other protein families and may be involved in self-association of the C1r and C1s within the Ca^{2+}-dependent $C1r_2$-$C1s_2$ complex, especially in view of the presence of β-hydroxyasparagine in this domain. The second set of repeating units located at the C-terminal ends of the C1r and C1s A chains are composed of the 60 amino acid short consensus repeats (SCRs) which are similar to the SCRs described in the C3b/C4b-binding proteins (discussed in Section 3.4) and which may play a role in the interaction of C1 with C4 or C2 (the substrates for activated C1s). The C1r and C1s genes are closely linked, being within 20 kb of each other on region p13 of human chromosome 12. It will be of interest, once the gene structures are available, to see if the various repeating units, growth factor-like domain and portions of the serine protease chain are precisely encoded by separate exons, as has been found to be the case for the factor B gene.

1.2 Factor D

Although early evidence for a precursor form of factor D has been further substantiated by cDNA cloning (4), it is still generally accepted that factor D circulates in the blood primarily in its active form. The requirement for activation of pro-enzyme D as an initial and limiting step in alternative pathway activation would appear to negate the large body of evidence supporting the view that alternative pathway activation is primarily dependent upon the preservation of the function of the C3b,Bb complex in 'protected sites' on an activator (Chapter 2, Section 3). Despite its high specificity for a single bond in factor B when in the C3b,B complex, factor D does not appear to have a large activation peptide or 'extension' to its serine protease domain (*Figure 3.1*). Biosynthetic studies and cDNA cloning indicates that D is encoded as a precursor of approximately 31 000 molecular weight (compared with a value of 25 000 for the serum enzyme), which would be consistent with a combined leader peptide plus precursor sequence of only 60 amino acids. Human factor D shows a remarkable 64% identity on alignment with mouse adipsin (a serine protease principally synthesized in adipose tissue and apparently involved in lipid metabolism). It also shows significant identity (>35%) on alignment with another principally intracellular protease—the rat mast cell protease II found in the granules of atypical mast cells. Factor D also appears to be the most closely related of the complement serine proteases to the family of serine proteases found in the granules of natural killer (NK) cells (see Section 5).

1.3 Factor B and C2

Despite the overall general similarity at the protein and mRNA levels between these two closely linked complement serine proteases, both encoded within the major histocompatibility complex (MHC) (5) (*Figure 3.2*), their genes differ considerably in size (factor B is 6 kb in size while C2 is 18 kb due to the presence of more intron sequences). The human factor B gene was the first complement gene to have its structure entirely determined (*Figure 3.2*) and certain interesting features with respect to the evolution and function of serine proteases have emerged from examination of the intron/exon boundaries of the gene. The 6 kb gene is split into 18 exons, the N-terminal Ba 'activation fragment' of 30 000 molecular weight being encoded by four exons (6). From the amino acid sequence data, it can be seen that Ba is composed of three 60 amino acid SCRs which are each precisely encoded by the three exons found after the exon encoding the leader sequence and a similar situation is probably true for the N-terminal portion of C2. Although the precise function of the 60 amino acid SCRs has not been established, they have been found in most of the complement proteins which interact with C3b or C4b (Section 4), and it seems likely that the Ba and C2b portions of factor B and C2 are directly involved in the initial binding to C3b and C4b, respectively, prior to the activation of factor B and C2, to form the C3 convertases (Chapter 2, Sections 1 and 3). The catalytic Bb peptide (60 000 mol. wt) is encoded by 13 exons and the amino acid sequences encoded by the first five of these exons show no homology with other serine proteases except C2. This would imply a role for the N-terminal portions of Bb and C2a in the interaction with C3b in the formation of the C3 and C5 convertase enzyme complexes. The C-terminal half of the Bb catalytic chain is homologous to the catalytic chains of other serine proteases, each of the functionally important parts of the active site being contained in separate exons. Thus, a close correlation with the exon organization of other serine proteases of the chymotrypsin/trypsin family is seen over this region with the exception of an 'extra' exon, exon 15, in factor B which has no counterpart except perhaps in the C2 gene (6). The role of the section of proteins encoded by this 'extra' exon may be to ensure that activated factor B cleaves only C3 and C5, or it may play a role in the manner in which the pro-enzyme is activated.

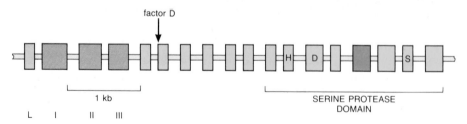

Figure 3.2.   Gene structure of human factor B. Exons are boxed. L encodes the majority of the leader peptide. Three SCRs are encoded by exons I – III. Exons containing active site residues [His (H), Asp (D) and Ser (S)] are indicated. The exon, shown in solid orange, is absent from other serine proteases (except C2) and may be important in conferring specificity.

1.4 Factor I

Factor I is synthesized as a single chain precursor of 88 000 mol. wt which is processed to yield the active form, composed of two disulphide-linked chains (50 000 and 38 000 mol. wts), found in plasma. Although factor I is resistant to one of the classical serine protease inhibitors (i.e. diisopropylphosphofluoridate) its amino acid sequence clearly shows that it belongs to the serine protease family (7). The amino acid sequence of the heavy chain is of a 'mosaic' nature, one striking feature being the presence of cysteine-rich units known as low density lipoprotein (LDL) receptor repeats class A and class B (EGF-like)—one class B repeat at position 12 – 59 and two class A repeats at positions 205 – 238 and 239 – 275. The presence of the class B repeats is seen in other complement proteins such as C1r and C1s and the terminal components (C7, C8α, C8β and C9) but the precise function of these units is unknown. They seem likely to play a role in the interaction of factor I with the C3/C5 convertases of either pathway of complement where it specifically splits the α' chains of the activation products (C4b and C3b) of components C4 and C3 in two or three positions, that is after association of the C4b or C3b with one of the appropriate cofactor proteins.

2. Class III gene products of the major histocompatibility complex (MHC)

The MHC is the name given to the genomic region where the transplantation antigens are coded. In man, it is located in the short arm of chromosome 6. It contains about 3.5×10^6 bp of genetic material. On the proximal end to the centromere, genes for the class II antigens are found. The distal end is marked by the genes for the heavy chain of the class I antigens (see *Figure 3.3*) (8). Both class I and class II antigens are membrane-bound proteins with the characteristic hydrophobic transmembrane segment. Whereas the class I antigens are ex-

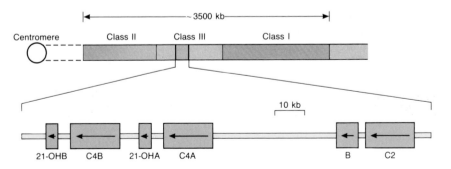

Figure 3.3.   MHC class III genes. A map of the human MHC (HLA) is shown above with class III genes lying between the class I and II regions. Within this region are the genes for the two isotypes of C4, the isotypes of the enzyme 21-hydroxylase (21-OHA and 21-OHB), factor B and C2, shown expanded below. Arrows indicate direction of transcription.

pressed on all nucleated cells, the class II antigens have a more select cellular and tissue distribution. The extracellular portions of both class I and class II antigens are composed of globular domains similar to those found on immunoglobulins. The class I and class II antigens serve as 'self' markers in the immune system. They play important roles in cell recognition so as to direct and regulate various activities of the cellular immune system to operate on the desired targets.

The region between class I and class II is defined as class III which spans approximately 1×10^6 bp of DNA. A 100 000 bp region containing the genes for three complement proteins (C2, C4, factor B) and the enzyme 21-hydroxylase has been well-characterized (5). The C2 and factor B genes are separated by less than 500 bp and the regulatory elements for factor B are actually found to overlap into the end of the C2 gene (9). The gene of factor B has been sequenced and is found to contain 18 small exons, with the three SCR units found in C3 and C4 binding proteins in three separate ones. The gene for C2 is about three times the size. Since the proteins are of similar sizes, the extra genetic material must be found in the non-coding regions. It remains a puzzle that this is not accounted for by the extra DNA found in one or a few introns, but by the increase of the average size of most introns. Both C2 and factor B are polymorphic but the number of common alleles are quite small (<5).

The class III region shown in *Figure 3.3* contains two C4 genes coding for the C4A and C4B isotypes, both of which function effectively as C4 in the complement system (10). This is not surprising since their amino acid sequences differ by less than 1%. However, they do have measurable differences in their covalent binding activities. C4A is about 100 times as efficient as C4B in reacting with amino groups, whereas it has only one-tenth the efficiency in reacting with hydroxyl groups. This is reflected in the lower specific haemolytic activity of C4A presumably because of its poor binding to the hydroxyl groups on the erythrocyte surface in the standard assay system (11,12). In general, C4A and C4B are also different in their antigenicity, with C4A carrying the blood group Rodgers antigen and C4B the Chido antigen, as well as in their electrophoretic mobility, with C4A being more anionic. However, this generalization breaks down when examined in detail (*Figure 3.4*) (13).

Perhaps because of the close proximity of the two genes and their extreme similarity, exchange of genetic information is frequent, leading to an array of C4 molecules with crossing-over properties. To date, there are about 35 allotypes of C4. The most common ones and their properties are set out in *Figure 3.4*. Genetic variation is also evident at the genomic level including deletions, duplications, C4B genes found in the C4A loci and vice versa, and genes not expressing a product (14). A list of these C4 gene structures, together with their approximate frequencies found in the Caucasoid population, is presented in *Figure 3.5*. The reason that these complement genes lie within the MHC is not known; it is possible that there is a selective advantage for linkage between particular sets of class I and II genes, and the class III genes have then become entrapped and maintained in the linkage group.

	C4A					C4B				
ALLOTYPE	A6	A4	A3	A2	A1	B5	B4	B3	B2	B1
Haemolytic activity	VL	L	L	L	L	H	H	H	H	H
Binding to – NH$_2$	+ + +	+ + +	+ + +	+ + +	+ + +	+	+	+	+	+
Binding to – OH	±	±	±	±	±	+	+	+	+	+
Antigenicity	Rg	Rg	Rg	Rg	Ch	Rg	Ch	Ch	Ch	Ch

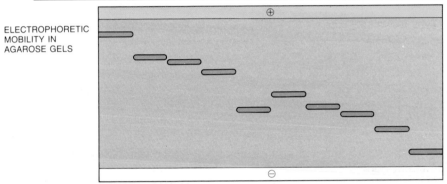

ELECTROPHORETIC
MOBILITY IN
AGAROSE GELS

Figure 3.4. Properties of common C4 allotypes. Haemolytic activity: H = high, L = low, VL = very low. C4A6 is very low since it cannot form a C5 convertase. Reactivity of binding to amino and hydroxyl groups is indicated between highly reactive (+ + +) and marginally reactive (±). Antigenicity: Rg = Rodgers, Ch = Chido. Note that C4A1 and C4B5 are atypical with respect to their antigenicity.

3. C3, C4 and C5

C3, C4 and C5 are synthesized as single polypeptides before they are secreted/processed, processes which include the removal of the signal peptide, glycosylation, sulphation, synthesis of the internal thiolester and the tailoring of the molecules by proteolysis of the single-chain pro-molecules to their final multi-chain structures. C3 and C4 each have an internal thiolester which is formed between the Cys residue and the Gln residue in a tetrapeptide, – Cys – Gly – Glu – Gln – (15). This thiolester is also found in the serum protease inhibitor α_2-macroglobulin (α_2M) and its related molecules, including the pregnancy zone protein (16). C5, which does not have the internal thiolester nor binds covalently to cell surfaces, was found to have the Cys replaced by a Ser, and the Glu by an Ala in the mouse protein. The structure of the thiolester site is shown in *Figure 3.6*. The activation of these molecules allows the thiolester to react with nucleophiles in the medium. In biological systems the most available nucleophiles are hydroxyl and amino groups. Interestingly, C3, the two isotypes of C4, C4A and C4B, and α_2M react differently with amino and hydroxyl groups (17). Since C4A and C4B only differ by four amino acid residues in their primary structure, it is reasonable to assume that these four residues must play a part in conferring

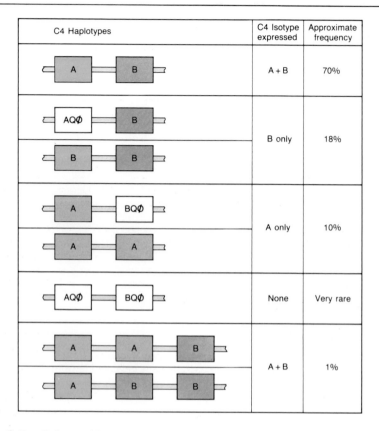

C4 Haplotypes	C4 Isotype expressed	Approximate frequency
A — B	A + B	70%
AQ∅ — B / B — B	B only	18%
A — BQ∅ / A — A	A only	10%
AQ∅ — BQ∅	None	Very rare
A — A — B / A — B — B	A + B	1%

Figure 3.5. Polymorphism of C4 gene expression. Genes in the C4A locus are in orange and genes of the C4B locus are brown. However, the gene type occupying this position and expressed is indicated by the letter on each gene locus. The haplotype frequency is typical for Caucasoid populations (adapted from ref. 4).

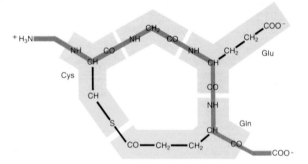

Figure 3.6. Chemical structure of the internal thiolester of C3 and C4. The 15-membered thiolactone ring is formed from four amino acid residues (backshaded orange), with a thiolester bond between Cys and Gln. The peptide backbone is in brown, side chains are black. The structure is conserved in all C3 and C4 molecules except mouse C4 which has Ala substituted for Gly.

Table 3.1. The reaction rates of glycine and glycerol with the thiolester-containing proteins

Proteins	Putative catalytic residues	Glycine	Glycerol
		$k'/k_0{}^b(M^{-1})$	
Human C4A	P C − − L D	13 400	1.3
Human C4B	L S − − I H	120	15.5
Human C3	D A − − I H	0	23.0
Human α_2M	S G − − L N	206	1.2
Mouse C4	P C − − I H	136	25.0

[a]The putative catalytic residues are at positions 1101, 1102, 1105 and 1106 of the human C4 sequences. The corresponding residues in C3, α_2-macroglobulin (α_2M) and mouse C4 are shown.
[b]The proteins are activated in the presence of radiolabelled glycine and glycerol. The exposed thiolester either reacts with the radioactive molecules or is hydrolysed by water. The fraction of protein bound with radioactive molecule is equal to $k'[G]/(k'[G] + k_0)$ where k' is the second order reaction rate of the protein with glycine or glycerol, k_0 is the rate of hydrolysis of the exposed thiolester, and $[G]$ is the concentration of glycine or glycerol in the reaction medium. The value k'/k_0 can be obtained accordingly.

specificity of the binding reaction. The reaction rates of the four proteins with amino and hydroxyl groups, and the four putative catalytic residues for each are shown in *Table 3.1*. The mechanism by which they confer specificity is not known.

The genes coding for C3, C4, C5 and α_2M are not linked. In man, the genes for C3 have been located on chromosome 19, C4 on chromosome 6 and α_2M on chromosome 12; that for C5 is not known. It could be argued that although they are likely to have evolved from an ancestral molecule and they share similarities in their structure and functions, they have diverged from each other to mediate their own specific activities. Separation of the genes may be a way to avoid unnecessary genetic events which could homogenize their structure and hence their functions.

4. Proteins interacting with C3b and C4b—relationship with the RCA gene cluster

A number of proteins associated with the complement system contain between two and 30 repeating units which have a similar (but not identical) structure of approximately 60 amino acids which conform to a consensus sequence repeat called an SCR. This has a framework of highly conserved residues involving one Trp, two Pro and four Cys residues, with conservation of Gly residues and hydrophobic residues at other positions (*Figure 3.7*). The determination of the precise boundaries of these tandem repeating structures is not always clear-cut at the protein level but studies at the gene level on a variety of the members of this group of proteins have shown that, in general, the SCRs can be defined

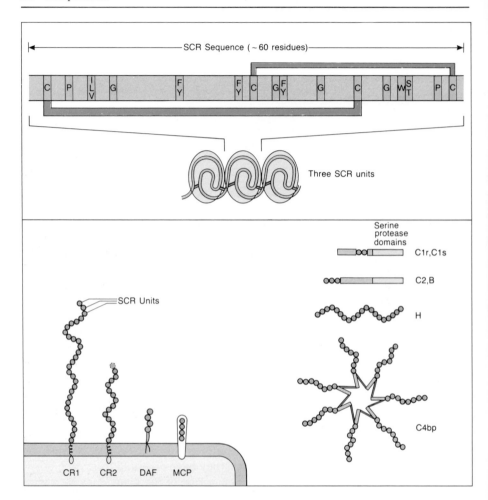

Figure 3.7.   Short consensus repeats. The schematic structure of SCRs is shown (top) consisting of approximately 60 amino acid residues, with two internal disulphide bonds (solid orange). Conserved residues are shown in shaded orange. These are thought to form small globular units, as indicated below, which are found in 10 complement proteins. At least three proteins outside the complement system are also found to contain SCR units.

by intron/exon boundaries, with each SCR being precisely encoded by separate exons. There are a few exceptions to this rule in some of the complement genes, with the second SCR of C4bp and the second SCR of H being encoded by two exons. The view that each SCR, as defined by primary and genomic structural analysis, represents individual domains in the protein structure is supported by the finding in at least three members of the group that the disulphide bonds appear to be arranged in a self-contained 1 – 3, 2 – 4 fashion, with no inter-SCR disulphide bonds being found to-date.

Family studies of the genes coding for the complement-associated SCR-containing proteins, either by allotypic polymorphism at the protein level or restriction fragment length polymorphism (RFLP) analysis at the nucleic acid level, have shown that the genes for CR1, factor H, C4 binding protein (C4bp) and decay accelerating factor (DAF) are closely linked and found on chromosome 1 in both mice and humans. This gene cluster is referred to as the RCA (regulators for complement activation) (18). Using pulsed-field electrophoresis, it has been found that a genomic fragment of 950 kb contained the genes for CR1, DAF and C4bp as well as CR2. The gene for factor H was not included in this fragment but it has been reported that the b chain of blood clotting factor XIII, a non-complement protein containing the SCRs, is linked to H and therefore is probably also within the RCA cluster. However, other complement proteins containing the SCRs are not linked to the RCA, with C2 and factor B being found on chromosome 6 and C1r and C1s on chromosome 12 in humans.

A feature which the complement-associated molecules, which contain the SCRs, have in common is that they show interaction with C4, C4b or C3b (except in the case of CR2 which shows affinity for C3dg). The significance of the SCRs in C3/C4-binding proteins is not certain and, although it is attractive to postulate that each SCR is a C3/C4-binding unit, with each unit contributing to the combined affinity of the protein for either C3 or C4, this view is not supported by the experimental data. For example, C4bp and factor H have specificities for C4 and C3 respectively, but cross-reactivities are very weak. Also, the cofactor activities of both H and C4bp are associated with particular (generally N-terminal) proteolytic fragments of the respective proteins. A number of non-complement proteins contain relatively large numbers of these SCRs (10 in the b chain of blood clotting factor XIII) and are not known to interact with C3 or C4. Thus, it is possible that the role of the SCRs is to confer a general structural framework that can be utilized in a variety of binding reactions in much the same way as the different immunoglobulin domains can fulfil a varied number of binding and functional roles.

The complement proteins with relatively few of the SCRs such as C1r, C1s and factor B and C2 seem most amenable to testing for function by modifying or replacing one particular SCR at a time. The pro-enzymes C1r and C1s each contain two SCRs, which suggests that eight SCRs could be aligned around the collagen-like cage of the C1q molecule in the $C1q-C1r_2-C1s_2$ complex, thus providing interaction with C4 prior to its activation. This would be consistent with several of the models proposed for the C1 complex (see Chapter 2, *Figure 2.2*) and should be quite readily testable. In the case of factor B and C2 it is well documented that the N-terminal C2b and Ba domains of these pro-enzymes, each containing three SCRs, associated with C4b and C3b, respectively, in a Mg^{2+}-dependent interaction. With respect to the proteins containing larger numbers of the SCRs, such as C4bp (56 SCRs), H (20 SCRs) and CR1 (30 SCRs), there is good evidence that only a limited number of the N-terminal SCRs are directly involved with C3b/C4b binding. Perhaps the C4bp molecule gives the clearest picture of the type of structure likely to be imparted to a plasma protein by the repeats. In the electron microscope C4bp appears as a spider-like structure with seven flexible 'tentacles' (each 3 nm × 33 nm) joined to a small central 'core' (*Figures 3.7 and 3.8*) (19). Each tentacle and one-seventh of the 'core' is

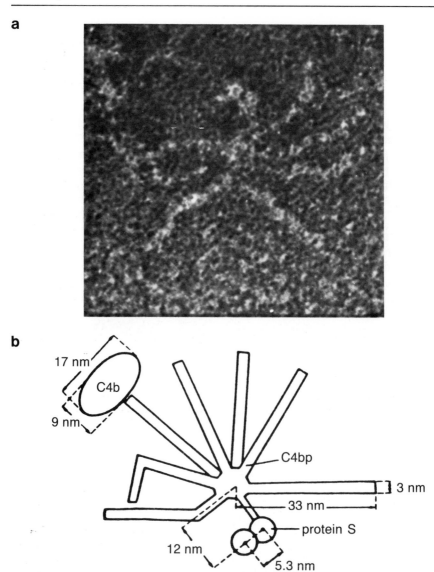

Figure 3.8. (a) An electron micrograph of C4b-binding protein showing its spider-like heptameric structure (kindly supplied by Dr B.Dahlbäck from ref. 19). **(b)** A schematic model of C4b-binding protein, complexed to C4b and to protein S, showing the relative dimensions of each of these molecules (from ref. 19).

considered to represent a chain of C4bp. The C-terminal 58 residues of each of the seven chains form a stable α-helical structure, disulphide-bonded core while the N-terminal 491 amino acids contain the eight SCRs which are formed predominately by β-sheets and random coils. It seems likely that the eight SCRs will form eight similar structural domains each of approximately 4 nm arranged

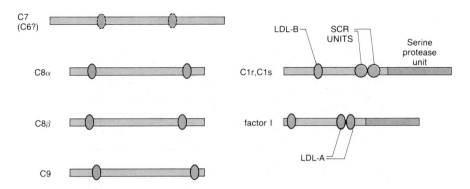

Figure 3.9. Cys-rich homologous structural units in complement proteins. These are of two types (LDL-A and LDL-B) based on their original discovery in LDL receptors. They occur in C1r, C1s, C7, C8, C9 and factor I. LDL-A units are orange ovals, LDL-B units are grey and SCR units are shown as orange discs.

in a linear and tandem fashion along the tentacle with the N-terminal SCR at the extremity. In the case of the membrane receptor CR1, except for the first two SCRs which may contain the C3b binding site, the remaining 28 SCRs may be simply playing a structural role to extend the binding site from plasma membrane so as to enhance its effectiveness.

5. The relationship between the terminal attack components and the perforins of killer lymphocytes

A striking feature of the terminal components of complement is the manner in which a group of soluble hydrophilic components (C5b, C6, C7, C8 and C9) rapidly undergo a hydrophilic – amphiphilic transition via a non-enzymatic, self-assembly, mechanism to form the membrane attack complex (MAC) containing up to 18 molecules of C9, which behaves as an integral membrane component.

It is clear that the C6, C7, C8α, C8β and C9 components of the MAC are structurally, antigenically and functionally related and comparison of their amino acid sequences shows 21 – 30% identity (20 – 22). All of the chains have a large internal domain which is almost free of Cys residues, an N-terminal domain which is homologous to the type A LDL receptor repeat and a C-terminal domain which is similar to the LDL receptor type B (EGF-like) repeat (*Figure 3.9*). For each of these proteins the N-terminal half is predominately hydrophilic in character while the C-terminal half contains several hydrophobic sections, which would be consistent, at least in the case of C9, with the view that the C-terminal half may be involved with insertion into the membrane. The presence of the 40 amino acids-long, Cys-rich LDL receptor type A receptor in N-terminal ends of C9, along with the finding that C9 polymerization can be inhibited by LDL, indicates that this Cys-rich domain in C9 may be of some functional importance in regulating the size of the MAC.

The formation of the MAC is similar in several respects to the Ca^{2+}-induced polymerization of perforin which is a 70 000 molecular weight glycoprotein present in the granules of cytotoxic T cells and NK cells (23). Purified perforin produces structural and functional lesions in target cells similar to those caused by intact killer cells or granules. An essential functional difference between C9 and perforin is that purified perforin will lyse erythrocytes and tumour cells in the presence of Ca^{2+} while C9 requires the prior assembly of C5b-8 on the target membrane before efficient cell lysis will take place. C9 also has the capacity to undergo a self-polymerization process yielding structures similar to poly-merized perforin, but this takes place under artificial laboratory conditions at high temperatures ($>37°C$) in the presence of high concentrations of Zn^{2+}. The sequence of the C-terminal region of mouse perforin shows 27% identity with the C-terminal region of C9, which includes complete identity of the six Cys residues of the EGF-like domain seen in C9.

Thus C6, C7, C8α, C8β, C9 and perforin appear to be both structurally and functionally related, suggesting that there is a family of such molecules involved in the disruption of invading organisms and perhaps tumour cells.

6. Complement receptor type 3 (CR3) and the leukocyte adhesion glycoproteins

C3b in serum is rapidly converted to iC3b by factor I and its cofactors. Even on activating surfaces of the alternative pathway where this conversion is retarded, a substantial level of iC3b is found. However, the subsequent digestion of iC3b to C3c and C3dg by serum proteases is relatively slow. Hence, the majority of bound C3 fragments on target surfaces is in the form of iC3b. It is therefore not surprising that a receptor specific for iC3b is required to partake in the elimination of opsonized targets. CR3 is found on phagocytes and its binding to iC3b requires divalent cations (24,25). Its role in phagocytosis, apart from its ligand specificity and cation requirement, is similar to that of CR1 (see Chapter 4, Section 4).

CR3 belongs to a group of three leukocyte surface antigens called the leukocyte adhesion glycoproteins, the other two being the lymphocyte-function-associated antigen 1 (LFA-1) and the p150,95 antigen (26). Each is composed of two non-covalently associated subunits; the α subunit is unique to each antigen but the β subunit is common. LFA-1 is found on lymphocytes and it mediates a wide range of T cell adhesion activities. p150,95 also binds iC3b and is speculated to be an alternative receptor for iC3b. In addition, the three antigens appear to have a broad range of binding activities with surface structures of micro-organisms, including bacterial lipopolysaccharides. Hence, they may be regarded as general receptors on leukocytes and one of the many ligands for two of them is iC3b (27,28).

The leukocyte adhesion glycoproteins are related to two other sets of cell surface antigens involved in cell adhesion activities. They are represented by the fibronectin receptor in one and the glycoprotein IIb/IIIa found on platelets in the other. The primary structures of their respective β subunits have recently become available and the polypeptides of the three β subunits show over 40% identity after alignment (29). The structure of the α subunit of CR3 is not known, but on the assumption that it is similar to that of p150,95, it could contain several calcium binding domains which may serve to account for its cation requirement for binding activities (30).

7. Variants on the typical complement proteins

The descriptions of complement proteins in this chapter are based on the properties of the most common forms present in blood and cell surfaces. It serves the purpose of illustrating the basic interactions between complement proteins and their coordinated activities in the elimination of invading micro-organisms. However, variations on the common forms do exist and some of them are discussed briefly in this section.

7.1 Polymorphism

Protein polymorphism is used to describe the minor variation in properties of a particular protein. Usually they are distinguished from each other by their mobility in an electric field, for example in agarose gel electrophoresis, or by their antigenicity. Most complement proteins are polymorphic, but in most cases their differences are not manifested at the functional level. However, by studying the polymorphism of the complement proteins in families, the genetic linkage between some of the components has been established.

The polymorphism in two complement proteins deserves separate attention: they are the plasma protein C4 and the membrane protein CR1. C4 is the most polymorphic among the complement proteins. To date, there are no less than 30 allotypes of C4 reported (31). The differences in their primary structure appear to be concentrated in the C4d region, conferring them with different electrophoretic and antigenic properties. As mentioned in Section 2, there are two C4 genes arranged in tandem in the human haploid genome. Usually, one codes for a C4A and the other for a C4B protein. The C4A and C4B proteins, since they are coded for by different genes, are the *isotypes* of C4. The properties of some of the most common C4A and C4B proteins are shown in *Figure 3.4*. Functionally, as measured by their haemolytic activity and covalent binding specificity with glycine and glycerol, all C4A allotypes have very similar, if not identical, properties and so have the C4B allotypes, although they differ from those of the C4A allotypes. Of specific interest is C4A6, which has very low haemolytic activity which was found to be caused by its inability to form an effective C5 convertase (32).

CR1 has a very unusual polymorphism which is related to the size of its polypeptide chain (33). The extracellular domain of CR1 appears to be composed entirely of SCR units and the most frequent CR1 allotype (CR1-A, frequency of 0.83) contains 30 SCR units (34). These 30 SCRs have a higher order of repeating structure in that the N-terminal 28 are arranged in four very homologous but not identical repeats, each containing seven SCRs. They are called long homologous repeats (LHRs) to be distinguished from the SCRs. Other allotypes are thought to differ from CR1-A and from each other by an integral number of LHRs. Thus CR1-B (frequency of 0.16) and CR1-C (frequency of 0.01) possibly have five LHRs (with 37 SCRs) and three LHRs (with 23 SCRs) respectively. This type of size variation, however, does not appear to affect the activity of CR1 as a regulatory protein.

7.2 Other variants

The structural variants of other complement proteins which are not considered to be hereditarily determined have been described. In most cases they are present in apparently normal individuals at low levels in comparison with the dominant forms, and they are encoded by different genes. These variants include the incompletely processed C4 (in that one of the chain junctions is not cleaved), the truncated versions of factor H and CR1, the high molecular weight (about twice as normal) forms of CR1 and DAF, the membrane-bound forms of factors H and B, and the soluble forms of CR1 and DAF. These proteins are not well characterized and their biological significance is not yet known.

8. Further reading

8.1 Molecular genetics of components of complement

Campbell,R.D., Carroll,M.C. and Porter,R.R. (1986) *Adv. Immunol.,* **38**, 203.
Campbell,R.D., Law,S.K.A., Reid,K.B.M. and Sim,R.B. (1988) *Annu. Rev. Immunol.,* **6**, 161.

8.2 The thiolester-containing proteins

Sottrup-Jensen,L. (1987) In Putnam,F.W. (ed.), *The Plasma Proteins.* Academic Press, Florida, Vol. V, p. 191.

8.3 Control proteins interacting with C3b and C4b

Reid,K.B.M., Bentley,D.R., Campbell,R.D., Chung,L.P., Sim,R.B., Kirstensen,T. and Tack,B.F. (1987) *Immunol. Today,* **7**, 230.

8.4 Relationship between terminal components and perforin

Müller-Eberhard,H.J., Zalman,L.S., Chin,F.J., Jung,G. and Martin,D.E. (1986) *Prog. Immunol.* **VI**, 268.
Young,J.D.E., Cohn,Z.A. and Podack,E.R. (1986) *Science,* **233**, 184.

8.5 C3 receptors

Fearon,D.T. and Wong,W.W. (1983) *Annu. Rev. Immunol.,* **1**, 243.
Hynes,R.O. (1987) *Cell,* **48**, 549.
Law,S.K.A. (1988) *J. Cell Sci.,* in press.
Sim,R.B. and Walport,M.J. (1987) In Whaley,K. (ed.), *Complement in Health and Disease.* MTP Press Ltd, Lancaster, p. 125.

8.6 C4 polymorphism

Porter,R.R. (1983) *Mol. Biol. Med.,* **1**, 161.
Sim,E. and Dodds,A.W. (1987) In Whaley,K. (ed.), *Complement in Health and Disease.*
   p. 99.

9. References

1. Neurath,H. (1984) *Science,* **224**, 350.
2. Journet,A. and Tosi,M. (1986) *Biochem. J.,* **240**, 783.
3. Tosi,M., Duponche,C., Meo,T. and Julier,C. (1987) *Biochemistry,* **26**, 8516.
4. Mole,J.E. and Anderson,J.K. (1987) *Complement,* **4**, 196.
5. Carroll,M.C., Campbell,R.D., Bentley,D.R. and Porter,R.R. (1984) *Nature,* **307**. 237.
6. Bentley,D.R. and Campbell,R.D. (1986) *Biochem. Soc. Symp.,* **51**, 7.
7. Catterall,C.F., Lyons,A., Sim,R.B., Day,A.J. and Harris,T.J.R. (1987) *Biochem. J.,*
    242, 840.
8. Dunham,I., Sargent,C.A., Trowsdale,J. and Campbell,R.D. (1987) *Proc. Natl. Acad.*
    Sci. USA, **84**, 7237.
9. Wu,L.C., Morely,B.J. and Campbell,R.D. (1987) *Cell,* **48**, 331.
10. Belt,K.T., Yu,C.Y., Carroll,M.C. and Porter,R.R. (1985) *Immunogenetics,* **21**, 173.
11. Law,S.K.A., Dodds,A.W. and Porter,R.R. (1984) *EMBO J.,* **3**, 1819.
12. Isenman,D.E. and Young,J.R. (1984) *J. Immunol.,* **132**, 3019.
13. Dodds,A.W., Law,S.K.A. and Porter,R.R. (1986) *Immunogenetics,* **24**, 279.
14. Hauptmann,G., Goetz,J., Uring-Lambert,B. and Grosshans,E. (1986) *Prog. Allergy,*
    39, 232.
15. Tack,B.F., Harrison,R.A., Janatova,J., Thomas,M.L. and Prahl,J.W. (1980) *Proc.*
    Natl. Acad. Sci. USA, **77**, 5764.
16. Sottrup-Jensen,L., Stepanik,T.M., Wierzbicki,D.M., Jones,C.M., Lønblad,P.B.,
    Kristensen,T., Mortensen,S.B., Peterson,T.E. and Magnusson,S. (1983) *Ann. N. Y.*
    Acad. Sci., **421**, 41.
17. Dodds,A.W. and Law,S.K.A. (1988) *Complement,* in press.
18. Rodrigues de Cordoba,S., Lublin,D.M., Rubinstein,P. and Atkinson,J.P. (1985)
    J. Exp. Med., **161**, 1189.
19. Dahlback,B., Smith,C.A. and Müller-Eberhard,H.J. (1983) *Proc. Natl. Acad. Sci.*
    USA, **80**, 3461.
20. DiScipio,R.G., Gehring,M.R., Podack,E.R., Kan,C.C., Hugli,T.E. and Fey,G.H.
    (1984) *Proc. Natl. Acad. Sci. USA,* **81**, 7298.
21. Stanley,K.K., Kocher,H.-P., Luzio,J.P., Jackson,P. and Tschopp,J. (1985) *EMBO*
    J., **4**, 375.
22. Howard,O.M.Z., Rao,A.G. and Sodetz,J.N. (1987) *Biochemistry,* **26**, 3565.
23. Tschopp,J., Masson,D. and Stanley,K.K. (1986) *Nature,* **322**, 831.
24. Wright,S.D. and Silverstein,S.C. (1982) *J. Exp. Med.,* **156**, 1149.
25. Ross,G.D., Newman,S.L., Lambris,J.D., Devery-Pocius,J.E., Cain,J.A. and
    Lachmann,P.J. (1983) *J. Exp. Med.,* **158**, 334.
26. Sanchez-Madrid,F., Nagy,J.A., Robbins,E., Simon,P. and Springer,T.A. (1983)
    J. Exp. Med., **158**, 1785.
27. Ross,G.D., Thompson,R.A., Walport,M.J., Springer,T..A., Watson,J.V., Ward,
    R.H.R., Lida,J., Newman,S.L., Harrison,R.A. and Lachmann,P.J. (1985) *Blood,* **66**,
    882.
28. Wright,S.D. and Jong,M.T.C. (1986) *J. Exp. Med.,* **164**, 1876.
29. Law,S.K.A. (1988) *J. Cell Sci.,* in press.
30. Corbi,A.L., Miller,L.J., O'Conner,K., Larson,R.S. and Springer,T.A. (1987)
    EMBO J., **6**, 4023.
31. Mauff,G., Alper,C.A., Awdeh,Z., Batchelor,J.R., Bertrams,T., Braun-Petersen,G.,
    Dawkins,P.L., Demant,P., Edwards,J., Grosse-Wilde,H., Hauptmann,G., Klonda,P.,

Lamm,L., Mollenhauer,E., Nerl,C., Olaisen,B., O'Neill,G.J., Rittner,C., Roos,M.H., Skanes,V., Teisberg,P. and Wells,L. (1983) *Immunobiology*, **164**, 184.

32.   Dodds,A.W., Law,S.K.A. and Porter,R.R. (1985) *EMBO J.*, **4**, 2239.

33.   Holers,V.M., Chaplin,D.D., Leykam,J.F., Gruner,B.A., Kumar,V. and Atkinson,J.P. (1987) *Proc. Natl. Acad. Sci. USA*, **84**, 2459.

34.   Klickstein,L.B., Wong,W.W., Smith,J.A., Weis,J.H., Wilson,J.G. and Fearon,D.T. (1987) *J. Exp. Med.*, **165**, 1095.

4

Role of complement in health and disease

1. Biosynthesis of complement components

Most of the soluble plasma complement proteins are synthesized in the liver. Membrane-bound control proteins, of course, are synthesized in the cells on which they are expressed. Extrahepatic synthesis of the soluble proteins, though accounting for a minority of the proteins in plasma, may be important in the secretion of these proteins locally. A case in point would be the synthesis and secretion of complement proteins by macrophages at sites of injury (1). The rate of complement turnover increases in conditions such as vasculitis associated with rheumatoid disease. However, increased catabolism is compensated for by increased synthesis, so that it is only in the most severe cases that total serum levels of components such as C3 are significantly depressed.

The synthesis and processing of complement proteins are no different from those of any other secreted and membrane proteins. Most components are single polypeptide chains. Some of them are synthesized as a single polypeptide and then processed into a multi-chain molecule such as C3, C4, C5 and factor I (2). In these four cases the processing requires the removal of four basic residues separating the chains in the pro-molecule, and it is likely to involve a mixture of enzymes with trypsin-like and carboxypeptidase activities. Some components are composed of more than one gene product, which combine to form a functional molecule such as in the case of C8, a complex of three gene products, and in the case of CR3, which is a complex of two. C4 binding protein (C4bp) and properdin (P) are oligomers of a single gene product. The most complicated of all is C1q, which contains six copies of each of three gene products. The 18 polypeptides combine to form a remarkable tulip-shaped molecule as shown by electron microscopy. The processing of pro-C4 to C4 is representative of the different processing reactions (*Figure 4.1*). The steps include the conversion of a single chain to a multi-chain molecule by the removal of stretches of tetrabasic residues, the tailoring of the polypeptide by the further removal of 22 amino acids at the C-terminal end of its α chain (3), the addition of carbohydrates and

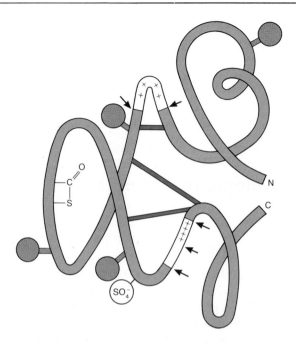

Figure 4.1.   The processing of C4. The single chain molecule of pro-C4 is processed by (i) the formation of the internal thiolester; (ii) the formation of disulphide bonds (solid orange); (iii) glycosylation (grey discs); (iv) sulphation, (v) the conversion to the three chain structure by removal of two stretches of tetrabasic residues (+ + + +); and (vi) the removal of 22 residues from the C-terminus of the α chain. Processing enzymes act on the unshaded areas of the pro-C4 chain at the places arrowed.

sulphates, the formation of disulphide bonds and the formation of the internal thiolester (4).

A most unusual structure found among the complement proteins is clearly the internal thiolester in C3 and C4. The glutamyl residue responsible for the carbonyl end of the thiolester is encoded as a glutamine residue. How the thiolester is formed between the sulphydryl of the Cys residue and the acylamino group of the Gln residue is not clear. Some preliminary data suggest that an enzyme may be required for the process. However, this enzyme has yet to be identified and isolated (5).

The level of each complement protein in plasma varies from the highest concentration found in C3 of about 1.3 g/l to the lowest in factor D at 1 mg/l. These levels are probably not arbitrary but represent a very delicately balanced composition of all the components in the system. The control elements in the genes for the complement proteins must play an important role in the regulation of the level of these components.

Modulators of complement levels include various hormones, lymphokines and endotoxins of bacterial origin, as well as one activation product of complement itself, C5a. This type of response may be of prime importance for phagocytic cells, whose synthesis and secretion of complement proteins at the site of inflammatory injury may play a direct role in the local clearance of infectious agents.

2. Immune complex clearance

Complement deficiences provide a strong clue to the possible role of complement in immune complex clearance. For deficiences of component C5 and upwards there is, in general, no impairment in the handling of immune complexes. However, there is a high incidence of immune complex disease in people having a homozygous deficiency of any of the early acting classical pathway components, that is C1q, C1r, C1s, C4, C2 and C3 (see Section 8). This is consistent with the finding that the classical pathway plays an important initial role in preventing the formation and precipitation of large immune complexes during the early stages of antibody – antigen interaction while the alternative pathway is important in solubilization of complexes once they are formed (*Figure 4.2*) (6 – 8). On interaction of serum antibodies with protein or particulate antigens a large lattice of interconnecting molecules can be formed due to the bivalency of IgG and multivalency of IgM antibody. The sizes of complex formed are highly dependent upon the ratio of antigen to antibody and once the complex reaches a certain size maximum precipitation occurs (when all the antibody has been precipitated this is known as the equivalence point). When antibody is in excess precipitation still occurs, but when antigen is in excess soluble complexes are formed. Studies carried out *in vitro* have shown that preformed immune complexes can be solubilized by the action of the alternative pathway components C3, B and D, which results in both the antigen and antibody in the complex becoming coated with C3b. For the effective deposition of C3b onto the complex, the presence of the control proteins, P, and factors H and I are required to prevent the loss of all the C3b in the fluid phase. After initial activation, assembly of $\overline{\text{C3b,Bb,P}}$ takes place on the complex, allowing generation and deposition of large numbers of C3b molecules, with approximately one molecule of C3b being bound per IgG. A significant portion of the bound C3b is located in the Fd region of IgG antibody (in the N-terminal half of the heavy chain, which partly contributes to the antigen binding site), which may be important in helping to disrupt the antibody – antigen lattice and also possibly interfering with Fc – Fc interactions which are considered to play a role in immune precipitation. The classical pathway appears to have a non-essential role in this solubilization process (as long as the aggregated antigen or antibody in the complex can act as an efficient alternative pathway activator) but would serve to accelerate and increase the efficiency of the reaction. However, *in vivo* it is probably of more physiological relevance that the formation of large immune complexes be prevented and *in vitro* studies have shown that significantly less C3b (~ one molecule per three IgG molecules) is required to prevent the initial formation and precipitation than is required for solubilization. It has been shown that activation of the classical pathway during formation of the immune complexes significantly delayed precipitation and the use of sera

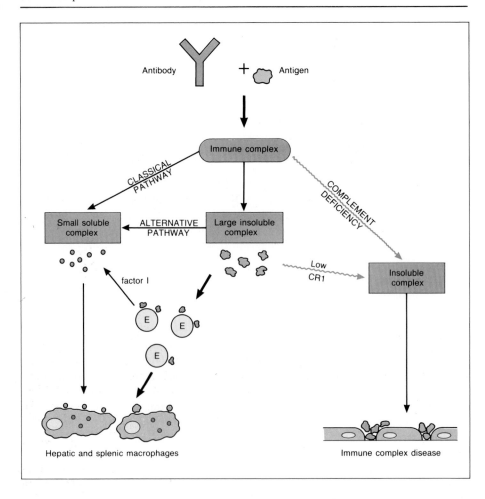

Figure 4.2.   The participation of complement in the handling of immune complexes (adapted from ref. 22). Small complexes are cleared by macrophages, large complexes will normally bind to erythrocytes (E) via CR1, but if CR1 is low or there is a complement deficiency (non-functional allotype, activation inhibitor etc.) insoluble complexes form.

depleted of B, D or P indicated that the alternative pathway was not required for this effect. A schematic drawing to scale of the interaction between immune aggregates and the early classical components is shown in *Figure 4.3*.

When considering immune complex disease in the general population then, of course, the majority of patients do not completely lack the early acting complement components. The types of immune complex disease are quite varied, for example rheumatoid arthritis (where an inflammatory response is brought about by presence of antibody – antigen complexes in the synovial fluid); types of glomerulonephritis (due to trapping of complex within the glomerulus or the binding of antibody to antigens in the glomerulus); extrinsic allergic alveolitis

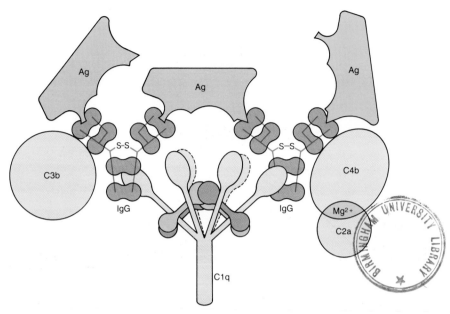

Figure 4.3. Interaction of the early classical complement components with antibody – antigen (Ag) complexes. Interaction of the C1 complex (C1q-C1r₂-C1s₂) with antibody IgG, by the binding of the heads of C1q to the C_H2 domain of the Fc region of the immunoglobulin, allows activation of the C1r and C1s proenzymes to take place. The activated C̄1s, in the bound C̄1 complex, continues activation by splitting C4 into C4b plus C4a which, in turn, leads to the formation of the C3 convertase and splitting of C3 into C3b and C3a (Section 2.2). A small percentage of the freshly activated C4b and/or C3b becomes covalently bound to the Fd regions (N-terminal halves of the heavy chains) of the antibody molecule—a process which may be of importance in the control of immune complex formation and elimination. Control of the activated C̄1 complex is mediated by C1-inhibitor which combines stoichiometrically with C̄1r and C̄1s, removing them from the antibody – antigen aggregate thus leaving the collagen-like regions of C1q free to interact with suitable receptors found on a wide variety of cells (*Table 1.3*).

(as in 'farmer's lung' where the antigens are inhaled); filariasis (where antigens may be released from parasites on the lymphatic vessels); and erythema nodosum leprosum (where chemotherapy of patients with high levels of antibody against the leprosy bacillus results in antigen release and immune complex formation). In these types of patients more subtle 'defects' of the complement system may play a role, for example the sera from individuals who lack the C4A isotype are less effective at keeping immune complexes in solution than those who lack the C4B isotype. This suggests the possible involvement of the covalent binding of C4b via amino groups in solubilizing complexes. Diseases which reduce complement levels may also contribute to immune complex formation. Likewise, conditions which raise levels of any serum proteins that can carry out an inhibitory role on the initial interaction of the classical pathway with immune complexes by binding to IgG, thus preventing C1 binding and activation, could predispose an individual to immune complex disease. It is also possible for pathological

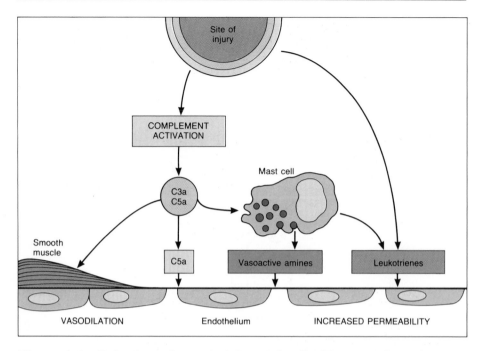

Figure 4.4. Role of complement in inflammation (I), C5a, vasoactive amines and leukotrienes act on endothelium to increase vascular permeability, while histamine and the anaphylatoxins act on smooth muscle of the vessel walls, to increase local blood supply.

events to exacerbate the effects of complement activation in immune complex disease. An example is the production of C3 nephritic factor (C3NeF) in some patients with membranoproliferative glomerulonephritis. C3NeF is an auto-antibody which binds to and stabilizes the alternative pathway C3 convertase, thereby potentiating C3 deposition on complexes in kidney gomeruli, via the alternative pathway. Once immune complexes are coated with C3b, they can be recognized by the CR1 receptor on red blood cells (9) and eliminated via cells of the monocyte/macrophage series in liver and spleen.

3. Inflammation

Tissue injury, if complicated by infection, triggers a set of reactions resulting in the migration of phagocytes to the site, accompanied by vasodilation, increase in blood supply and increased capillary permeability. Activation of the complement system by an infectious agent causes the release of three anaphyla-toxins, C4a, C3a and C5a, from their parent molecules (10). They are very similar in structure and mediate a similar set of activities but with different efficiencies (C5a > > C3a > > C4a). The anaphylatoxins induce vasodilation, but the same effect is probably amplified by vasoamines, the major one being histamine, which

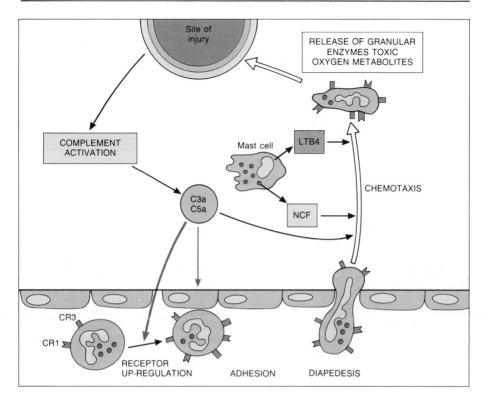

Figure 4.5.   Role of complement in inflammation (II). C3a and C5a enhance expression of complement receptors CR1 and CR3 on phagocytes and promote adhesion to endothelium. They also trigger mast cells to release neutrophil chemotactic factor (NCF) and synthesize leukotriene B4 (LTB4). These factors and C5a are chemotactic.

are released by mast cells under the stimulation of the anaphylatoxins. A direct consequence of vasodilation is the increase in local blood supply. The stress on the endothelial cells lining the blood vessel also allows plasma proteins to diffuse out of the blood vessel to the site of injury (*Figure 4.4*). This, of course, could be viewed as a positive feedback to increase the local level of complement proteins. The action of triggering mast cell degranulation requires the C-terminal Arg residue in the anaphylatoxins. Removal of the Arg by the anaphylatoxin inactivator (carboxypeptidase N) abolishes their capacity to bind to receptors on mast cells. Thus, the inflammatory process is localized to the primary site of injury.

C5a is the principal chemotactic factor for phagocytes, although C3a may have significant, but much lower, activity. In contrast to its effect on mast cells, the removal of Arg from the C-terminal of C5a only partially reduces its capacity as a chemotactic factor. Migration of C5a into the blood stream could also be assisted by vasodilation. The binding of C5a to blood phagocytes causes them to adhere to the endothelial cells lining the blood vessel, followed by their infiltration through the basement membrane and their chemotaxis towards the site of injury up a concentration gradient of C5a. A set of cellular responses is also evident: (i) an internal pool of complement receptors, both CR1 and CR3, and possibly the p150,95 antigen, are mobilized to the cell surface, and this could be the direct cause of the adherence of phagocytes to the endothelium (other studies have implicated that p150,95 is the mediator of neutrophil traffic into tissues); (ii) the release of intracellular enzymes and leukotrienes; and (iii) the production of toxic oxygen metabolites. Each of these responses could be considered as an enhancement of the cytotoxic capacity of the phagocytes. The activities of the anaphylatoxins on phagocyte cells are illustrated in *Figure 4.5*.

4. Opsonization and phagocytosis

Phagocytes, whose function is to ingest and dispose of unwanted cell debris, immune aggregates, bacteria and other micro-organisms, can only do so if they can recognize and distinguish them from host cells. The host defence therefore labels these targets with antibody and complement fragments, and the phagocytes recognize these labels by the specific receptors on their membrane surface. The coating of targets with antibody and complement fragments is frequently referred to as 'opsonization', which means 'preparation for food'.

Phagocytes include the polymorphonuclear leukocytes and monocytes in the blood and cells of the macrophage/monocyte lineage in various tissues and organs. The phagocytic receptors are the Fc receptors, which recognize the Fc portion of the antibody, and CR1 and CR3, which recognize C3b and iC3b, respectively.

The interaction of Fc receptor and antibody is sufficient to trigger the ingestion process provided the level of antibody on the targets is high enough to initiate efficient binding of phagocytes. A low level of antibody on the targets, which may not promote binding of phagocytes effectively, could activate the complement pathway. The deposition of C4 and C3 fragments on the targets amplifies the opsonic signal of the antibody, thus enhancing the efficiency of phagocyte binding via the complement receptors. The interaction between the complement receptors and C3 fragments does not necessarily trigger the ingestion process. In some cases, the interaction merely initiates the binding between phagocytes and targets to allow effective interaction between antibody and the Fc receptor. In other cases, the interaction itself is sufficient to promote the entire phagocytic event. The molecular nature of this distinction is not clear, though it has been speculated that phosphorylation of the receptors may promote them to the active state (11).

Interaction of ligand with receptors must generate a signal to the phagocyte to proceed with the ingestion process. The details of the communication are not known but it must ultimately be relayed to the actin network in the cytoskeleton since treatment of phagocytes with drugs known to disrupt actin filaments (e.g. cytochalasin B) inhibits the ingestion phase of phagocytosis, although the adherence of opsonized targets to phagocytes remains unimpaired (12).

After ingestion, the resultant internalized vesicles, called phagosomes, are

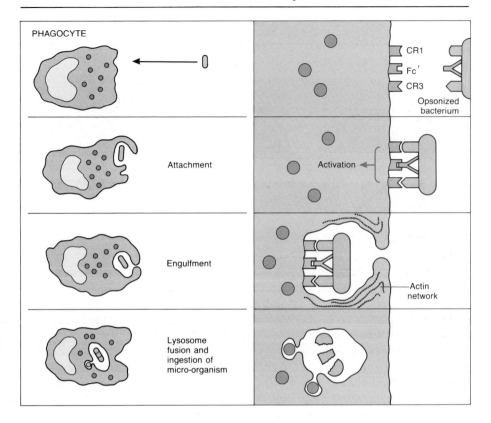

Figure 4.6. Opsonization and phagocytosis. Opsonized particles attach to phagocytes via CR1, CR3 and Fc receptors (Fc^r). Binding activates oxidative killing mechanisms, and the actin network to cause engulfment of the particle. The internalized material is attacked by reactive oxygen intermediates and by lysosomal enzymes.

fused with lysosomes where the final act of eliminating the opsonized target is carried out by the lysosomal enzymes (*Figure 4.6*).

5. Lytic function

Usually the general concept of the lytic function of complement is equated to the type of membrane attack complex (MAC) lesions seen in a model system such as the lysis of IgM-antibody-coated red blood cells with a heterologous complement. This type of study, along with studies on the lysis of re-formed red blood cell 'ghosts' and artificial liposome structures, has clearly shown that a spectrum of C5b-8, C9$_n$-type complexes can be formed, which vary in the number of C9 molecules present, n lying between one and 18. A MAC pore diameter of about 10 nm can be seen when 15–17 C9 molecules are present, while an apparent pore size of ~3 nm has been estimated for a C5b-8(C9)$_2$

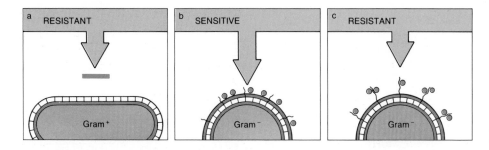

Figure 4.7. Sensitivity of bacteria to complement MAC. (**a**) Most Gram⁺ bacteria lack an outer lipid membrane and resist attack. (**b**) Some Gram⁻ bacteria are susceptible to the lytic components (orange discs) but some strains decoy the complement attack by producing long antigenic filaments which cause deposition away from the outer membrane (**c**).

complex, and it is considered that the smaller pores will fulfil a lytic function. However, some of the views concerning the mode of action may have to be modified with respect to the finding that nucleated cells appear to be capable of utilizing several defence mechanisms to escape MAC attack. It is known that in these cells there is a rise in the concentration of intracellular free calcium ions before any cell lysis becomes detectable, and that this can activate certain cellular functions which can cause either shedding or internalization of the MAC channels and perhaps the induction of lipid repair mechanisms, thus conferring protection. Unlike a red blood cell, which probably relies only on the binding of C9 by the homologous restriction factor (Chapter 2, Section 6.3) to inhibit attack by its own MAC, the nucleated cell is relatively resistant to complement. However, in the case of extensive complement activation ($\sim 10^5$ MACs/cell) even a nucleated target cell is unlikely to survive since early pore formation by the MAC would be accompanied by the breakdown of membrane potential, with a loss of potassium and influx of sodium. The subsequent compensatory ion-pumping mechanisms along with the cell activation induced by the rise in intra-cellular calcium may drain the cell of energy resources and this, along with the general marked physical alteration to the cell surface, is likely to promote cell death. In the case of the killing of Gram-negative bacteria, although initial complement activation may take place by either pathway, there is an absolute requirement for antibody to promote extensive complement activation and lysozyme also plays an important accessory role by attacking the peptidoglycan layer via the pores created by the MAC in the outer membranes. However, as in the case of nucleated cells, micro-organisms have evolved a variety of mechanisms by which they can prevent opsonization and lysis by complement, and this is emphasized by the finding that pathogenic bacteria isolated from patients often exhibit increased resistance to complement. Indeed, all Gram-positive bacteria are resistant, probably as a consequence of their thick peptido-glycan layer preventing access of C5b-9 to the minor membrane, and nearly all fungi resist complement attack by virtue of their rigid, relatively impermeable cell wall. Some strains of Gram-negative bacteria appear to be resistant to MAC attack by limiting complement activation to a subset of lipopolysaccharide molecules bearing longer than normal *O*-polysaccharide side chains, thus sterically hindering the C5b-9 complexes from reaching the complement-sensitive sites on the outer membrane (*Figure 4.7*).

Activation of complement to the C5b-9 stage is generally beneficial to the host in fighting infection but in certain disease states, especially those of an auto-immune nature, there may be damage of host cells and tissues. For example, kidney damage in systemic lupus erythematosus (SLE) and glomerular nephritis has been partly attributed to the MAC, as has injury to motor end plates in myasthenia gravis and to the muscular microvasculature in dermatomyositis. It is possible that apart from membrane damage, sublytic doses of the MAC may cause the release of toxic oxygen metabolites and arachidonic acid derivatives which may be involved in the pathogenesis of these conditions. These examples serve to emphasize the importance of mechanisms by which host cells may avoid damage by their own complement system.

6. General aspects of complement interaction with bacteria, parasites and viruses

The complement system is remarkable in that it can attach its activated components to, and attack, a wide variety of surfaces via hydroxyl or amino groups (covalently, through activated C4 and C3) or via membrane phospholipids through the MAC. This is amply demonstrated by considering the possible role of complement in the destruction and/or clearance of a wide variety of organisms such as Gram-negative and Gram-positive bacteria, parasites and viruses. Specificity and recognition of these interactions is often, but not always, a function of antibody binding which usually leads to efficient complement activation.

6.1 Bacteria

Complement was first described on the basis of its heat-sensitive bactericidal effect (*Figures 4.7* and *4.8*). Indeed, most Gram-negative bacteria can activate complement by both the classical and alternative pathways in the absence of antibody but efficient bacteriolysis of certain forms (the S forms) requires the bacterium to be coated with antibody. In the absence of antibody it is probably the lipopolysaccharide portion of the outer bacterial membrane which interacts directly with C1 to cause classical pathway activation and also provides a 'protected site' for the deposition of C3b, allowing formation of $\overline{\text{C3b,Bb}}$ and its protection from the effects of factors I and H, thus allowing efficient alternative pathway activation. The membranes of complement-sensitive Gram-negative bacteria display the same type of MAC lesions as those seen in the membranes of complement-lysed red blood cells. Intact Gram-positive bacteria, on the other hand, do not activate the classical pathway in the absence of antibody, which is probably due to the quite different cell wall composition of the two classes

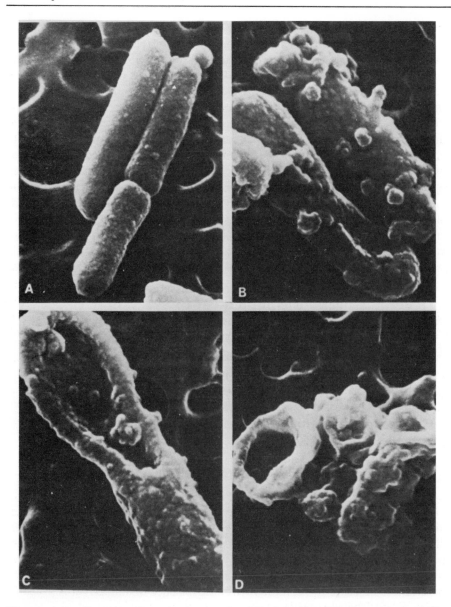

Figure 4.8.   Scanning electron micrographs of *Escherichia coli* before and after killing by complement (via the alternative pathway). **(A)** Intact bacteria. **(B and C)** Bacteria killed by mixture of purified alternative pathway complement components in the absence of lysozyme. Note the surface expansion and disruption of the membrane. **(D)** In the presence of both complement and lysozyme the cell damage is considerably increased (from ref. 23).

of bacteria. However, direct activation of the alternative pathway by Gram-positive bacteria does take place, as does activation of both pathways in the presence of the binding of specific antibodies. In all cases of complement activation, lysis of the Gram-positive bacteria does not take place but the bacteria become heavily coated with C3b and iC3b, allowing opsonization (see Section 4) of the bacteria by phagocytic cells. This is an important protective mechanism against both Gram-positive and Gram-negative bacteria and is well-illustrated by the sensitivity of C3-deficient individuals to bacterial infection.

Thus, it is now recognized that the composition of the bacterial envelope is important in determining sensitivity to the lytic action of complement, with Gram-negative bacteria usually being susceptible while Gram-positive bacteria are not. The composition of the bacterial membrane determines which complement pathway will be efficiently activated. It should also be noted that the surface composition of bacteria can be changed by plasmid-coded proteins which can induce resistance to complement lysis. In all cases the activation of complement leads to the opsonization of the bacteria.

6.2 Parasites

In view of the numerous different types of parasite it is difficult to form a general overview on the possible role of complement against infection by these organisms. One feature which emerges is that many parasites appear to activate the alternative pathway of complement, and this of course would be amplified by the presence of specific antibodies. Certainly, flagellates such a *Leishmania* and amoebae such as *Entamoeba histolytica* show sensitivity to complement, although in the case of *Schistosomes* complement appears to offer very little defence to infection. In certain cases complement may even provide beneficial effects to the parasites, for example by allowing entry into host cells of C3b- and/or iC3b-coated parasites (*Barbesia* and *Leishmania*) via CR1 and/or CR3 on host cells. Also, side effects due to activation of complement by immune complexes can lead to host problems, such as nephritis in malaria.

6.3 Viruses

Complement appears to play an important role in neutralizing viruses once the system has been activated by specific anti-viral antibodies. However, both pathways can also be triggered directly by viruses and virally infected cells without the aid of antibody. Direct activators of the classical pathway are the retroviruses Sindbis and Newcastle disease viruses, and activators of the alternative pathway are Epstein–Barr virus (EBV) and Sindbis virus. Antibody-independent activation of the alternative pathway is shown by cells infected with measles and EBV viruses. Although there is no definitive evidence that the action of complement plays a major role in the recovery from viral infection it certainly appears to play an accessory role to the mechanisms of anti-viral immunity. The coating of virus particles with C4b and C3b would be expected to prevent the virus from attaching to virus cell surface receptors and to prepare the virus for phagocytosis. Perhaps, on considering its possible role in the absence of antibody, complement could be viewed as being the humoral equivalent of the natural killer cell system, that is a humoral system which would provide some initial protection prior to the mounting of botn a humoral and a cellular immune response to a viral infection.

7. Possible role of complement in the immune response

Clearly defined roles in the immune response for the various complement components and fragments of the components, cannot be readily identified. However, it is becoming increasingly apparent that the complement system has the potential to interact with and modify the immune response at a number of steps: by the interaction with the various complement receptors for C3 and fragments of C3, such as CR1, CR2 and CR3; receptors for other complement components such as the H receptor and the C1q receptor found in a wide variety of lymphoid cells and, in certain cases, B and T cells (see *Table 1.3*); by the ability of the immunologically important lymphocytes and macrophages to synthesize C3 and a number of the other complement components (see Section 1); and by the regulation of lymphokine levels by a number of components and activated fragments of components. Another strong indicator of complement involvement with the immune response are the findings that human C4 deficiency and guinea pig C4 and C2 deficiencies appear to be associated with depression of the immune response (13,14).

Early *in vivo* studies using animals treated with cobra venom factor (CVF), which greatly reduces complement levels, indicated that complement might play a role in the immune response (15) since marked effects such as inhibition of primary and secondary T-dependent antibody responses were demonstrated. The protein in CVF which reduces complement levels is cobra C3b which forms an efficient and stable C3 convertase (CVF,Bb,P) in mammalian sera and is not susceptible to control by the action of factors I and H. Although the primary effect of CVF is to dramatically reduce C3 levels, the fact that CVF causes a continuous rapid activation and turnover of the alternative pathway made interpretation of these *in vivo* results difficult. Subsequent *in vivo* work has centred around the use of C3, fragments of C3 and antibodies to C3 to modify the immune response. These studies indicated that: (i) $F(ab')_2$ anti-C3 could inhibit primary and secondary T-dependent antibody production; (ii) C3a can inhibit B cell responses via the production of prostaglandins (however, on loss of its C-terminal Arg, C3a is inactive, and this happens very quickly in the blood, see Chapter 2, Section 6.2); (iii) C3d-K (a kallikrein cleavage fragment of iC3b) acts as an inhibitor of mitogen-induced B and T cell proliferation; and (iv) aggregated C3b or C3d can regulate the growth of activated B cells by promoting the entry of the B cells into S phase thus enhancing division (however, soluble C3d can inhibit this process, suggesting that the effect seen with aggregated material may correspond to effects mediated by C3b or C3d on a surface, while the effect seen with the soluble material may reflect the action of fluid phase complement activation) (16,17). Although these studies indicate a close involvement of C3 and its receptors with the immune response, the studies on human patients deficient in C3 are equivocal. These patients do have recurrent severe infections but these appear to be primarily as a result of deficiencies in opsonization, bactericidal activity, immune adherence and chemotaxis since, in general, their immune response seems normal. A more striking effect on the immune response is noted in certain complement-deficient animals since the primary antibody response in C2- or C4-deficient guinea pigs is clearly depressed and repeated immunization fails to increase the response or switch the antibody isotype from IgM to IgG. It was further found that this depression of the immune response is probably due to the lack of activation of C3 via the classical pathway. Thus, although C3 may not be required for an immune response to take place, its activation products do play a role up- or down-regulating the response and in the maturation of the immune response.

Other components besides C3 which may play a role in regulating the immune response are C1q, C5 and perhaps factor H. It has been shown that binding of C1q, via its collagen-like 'stalks', to the C1q receptors on lymphoblastoid cells inhibits the interleukin-1-like activity which is constitutively produced by these cells and consequently could block interleukin-1-induced lymphocyte proliferation. On the other hand, the anaphylatoxin C5a (with or without its C-terminal Arg) has been shown to stimulate monocyte production of interleukin 1 and also to enhance antibody formation *in vitro*.

Clearly, future studies involving the use of highly purified components, perhaps generated by recombinant DNA techniques, and modified fragments or components are required to assess the precise role complement plays in regulating the immune response.

8. Complement deficiencies

Deficiencies in a number of complement proteins have been reported and patients suffer from various degrees of illness. The deficiencies can be roughly categorized into six groups: (i) the early classical pathway components; (ii) the alternative pathway components; (iii) C3; (iv) the components of the MAC; (v) the control proteins; and (vi) the receptors. A list of these deficiencies together with their associated major clinical symptoms can be found in *Table 4.1*.

General association can be found between the complement deficiencies and the clinical conditions of the patients in the first four groups. Conclusions can therefore be drawn with regard to the function and importance of different complement components or pathways *in vivo*. The classical pathway is required in the clearance of immune complexes since deficiencies in any of the components results in the common manifestation of immune complex disorders. It should be emphasized that in the case of C4, immune complex disorder is exclusively correlated with the deficiency of the C4A isotype, even at the level of heterozygous deficiency (18). Deficiencies in the alternative pathway components are rather rare, perhaps for the reason that they are usually fatal; there is no known factor-B-deficient person alive and there is only one case of partial deficiency in factor D, with recurrent infection as the major clinical problem. Deficiencies in the terminal complex components are correlated with susceptibility to recurrent neisserial infection (19) possibly because of the ability of these micro-organisms to survive as intracellular parasites in phagocytes. Thus, the lytic arm of the complement system is required for their clearance. Individuals

Table 4.1.   Complement deficiencies

Protein	Remarks	Relative frequencies[a]	Major clinical disorder	Minor clinical disorder
Classical complement components				
C1q		medium	immune complex diseases	recurrent infection
C1r		low	SLE, glomerulonephritis	recurrent infection
C1s		low	SLE	
C4		medium	immune complex diseases	recurrent infection
C2		high	SLE	recurrent infection
Alternative pathway components				
B	very rare	low	(may be fatal)	
D		low	recurrent upper respiratory infection	
P		low	severe meningitis	
C3				
C3		medium	recurrent infection	immune complex disease
Membrane attack complex				
C5		medium	recurrent neisserial infection	SLE
C6		medium	recurrent neisserial infection	SLE
C7		medium	recurrent neisserial infection	SLE
C8		medium	recurrent neisserial infection	SLE
C9	good health	very high		
Control proteins				
C1-Inh	low C4 and C2 levels	very high	Angiooedema	
Factor I	low C3 and factor B levels, no alternative pathway activity	low	recurrent infection	SLE
Factor H	partial (10%)	low	haemolytic uraemic syndrome	
Membrane proteins				
CR1[b]		medium	immune complex disorder	
CR3	defective in β-subunit, patients also deficient in LFA-1 and p150,95		recurrent pyogenic infection	
DAF[c]			paroxysmal noctural haemoglobinuria	

[a]The levels are arbitrarily denoted as low (<10), medium (10–15), high (50–250) and very high (>250) according to the number of cases reported. The numbers are partly based on a report in ref. (24). These data are intended to give relative frequencies among the complement deficiencies.
[b]May not be a true deficiency. Level of erythrocyte CR1 may be regulated by closely linked genetic element. Low level of CR1 may also be acquired in patients with SLE, rheumatoid arthritis, auto-immune haemolytic anaemia, AIDS and paroxysmal noctural haemoglobinuria.
[c]Probably not hereditary.

deficient in C9, however, are mostly healthy. This suggests that the four components, C5 – C8, are sufficient to cause significant membrane damage and cell death. Deficiencies in the control proteins usually result in the consumption of the complement components which are normally protected from non-specific activation. Deficiency in the C1-inhibitor (C1-Inh) allows C1s to deplete C4 and C2 levels in serum and it is believed that hereditary angiooedema, generally associated with C1-Inh deficiency, could be caused by the increase of a C2 breakdown product. Deficiency in factor I allows the alternative pathway to accelerate into the positive feedback loop in the fluid phase, thus depressing the level of both factor B and C3 (20). These patients generally suffer from bacterial infections due to lack of opsonization brought about by freshly activated C3. Deficiencies in factor H and decay accelerating factor are less damaging clinically, since their functional activities are also mediated by other molecules, for example CR1. Deficiency in CR3 is always accompanied by the deficiency of two other proteins, p150,95 and LFA-1, because all patients identified to date have a defective gene for the β subunit. Patients with CR3 deficiency suffer from general recurrent infections, thus emphasizing the importance of the opsonic clearance of infectious micro-organisms (21).

9. Further reading

9.1 Immune complex clearance

Whaley,K. (ed.) (1987) In *Complement in Health and Disease*. MTP Press, Lancaster, p. 163.

9.2 Inflammation

Springer,T..A. and Anderson,D.C. (1986) In Kay,J., Kerr,M.A., Williams,A.F. and Reid,K.B.M. (eds) *Genes and Proteins in Immunity*. University Press, Cambridge, p. 47.

9.3 Anaphylatoxins and receptors

Huey,R., Fukuoka,Y., Hoeprich,P.D.,Jr and Hugli,T.E. (1986) In Kay,J., Kerr,M.A., Williams,A.F. and Reid,K.B.M. (eds), *Genes and Proteins in Immunity*. University Press, Cambridge, p. 69.

9.4 Opsonization

Ross,G.D. (ed.) (1986) In *Immunobiology of the Complement System*. Academic Press, New York, p. 87.

9.5 Complement and immune response

Weiler,J.M. (1987) In Whaley,K. (ed.), *Complement in Health and Disease*. MTP Press, Lancaster, p. 289.

9.6 Complement deficiency

Colten,H.R. (1986) *BioEssays*, **4**, 249.
Lachmann,P.J. and Walport,M.J. (1986) In Ross,G.D. (ed.), *Immunobiology of the Complement System*. Academic Press, New York, p. 237.
Thompson,R.A. (1987) In Whaley,K. (ed.), *Complement in Health and Disease*. MTP Press, Lancaster, p. 37.

10. References

1. Ezekowitz,R.A.B., Sim,R.B., Hill,H. and Gordon,S. (1984) *J. Exp. Med.,* **159**, 244.
2. Campbell,R.D., Law,S.K.A., Reid,K.B.M. and Sim,R.B. (1988) *Annu. Rev. Immunol.,* **6**, 161.
3. Law,S.K.A. and Gagnon,J. (1985) *BioSci. Rep.,* **5**, 913.
4. Karp,D.R. (1983) *J. Biol. Chem.,* **258**, 14490.
5. Iijima,M., Tobe,T., Sakamoto,T. and Tomita,M. (1984) *J. Biochem.,* **96**, 1539.
6. Schifferli,J.A., Wood,P. and Peters,D.K. (1982) *Clin. Exp. Immunol.,* **47**, 555.
7. Takata,Y., Tamura,N. and Fujita,T. (1984) *J. Immunol.,* **132**, 2531.
8. Schifferli,J.A., Ng,N.C. and Peters,D.K. (1986) *N. Eng. J. Med.,* **315**, 488.
9. Schifferli,J.A. and Peters,D.K. (1983) *Clin. Exp. Immunol.,* **54**, 827.
10. Hugli,T.E. (1985) In Müller-Eberhard,H.J. and Miescher,P.A. (eds), *Complement.* Springer-Verlag, Berlin, p. 73.
11. Wright,S.D. and Detmers,P.A. (1988) *J. Cell Sci.,* in press.
12. Axline,S.G. and Reaven,E.P. (1974) *J. Cell Biol.,* **62**, 647.
13. Sjoholm,A.G., Hammarstrom,L., Smith,C.I.E. and Kjellman,N.I.M. (1985) *Acta Pathol. Microbiol. Immunol. Scand., Series C,* **93**, 169.
14. Botteger,E.C., Hoffmann,T., Hadding,U. and Bitter-Suerman,D. (1985) *J. Immunol.,* **135**, 400.
15. Pepys,M.B. (1976) *Transplant. Rev.,* **32**, 93.
16. Erdei,A., Melchers,F., Schulz,T. and Dierich,M. (1985) *Eur. J. Immunol.,* **15**, 184.
17. Melchers,F., Erdei,A., Schulz,T. and Dierich,M. (1985) *Nature,* **317**, 264.
18. Fielder,A.H.L., Walport,M.J., Batchelor,J.R., Rynes,R.I., Black,C.M., Dodi,I.A. and Hughes,G.R.V. (1983) *Brit. Med. J.,* **286**, 425.
19. Peterson,B.H., Lee,T.J., Snyderman,K. and Brooks,G.F. (1979) *Annu. Intern. Med.,* **90**, 917.
20. Davis,A.E.,III, Davis,J.S.IV., Robson,A.R., Osofsky,S.G., Colten,H.R., Rosen,F.S. and Alper,C.A. (1977) *Clin. Immunol. Immunopathol.,* **8**, 543.
21. Anderson,D.C. and Springer,T.A. (1987) *Annu. Rev. Med.,* **38**, 175.
22. Whaley,K. (ed.) (1987) In *Complement in Health and Disease.* p. 175.
23. Schreiber,R.D., Morrison,D.C., Podack,E.R. and Müller-Eberhard,H.J. (1979) *J. Exp. Med.,* **149**, 870.
24. Schifferli,J.A. and Peters,D.K. (1983) *Lancet,* **ii**, 957.

5

Conclusion

The complement proteins, of both the soluble and membrane-bound types, form an effector arm of the humoral immune system. Normally passive, they can be activated when challenged by the invasion of a foreign object, for example in the form of an infectious micro-organism, via either an antibody-dependent (classical) or an antibody-independent (alternative) pathway. Activation involves a combination of limited but specific proteolysis of some components and induced conformational change in others. The molecular interactions in the activation steps leading to the elimination of the foreign object are described in Chapter 2. To function effectively and efficiently, the overall activity of complement has to be both non-specific, in that it has to be effective against a wide range of infectious micro-organisms, and specific, in that the incidental damage incurred to host cells and tissues in the elimination of the infectious micro-organisms has to be kept to a minimal level. These two criteria can be appreciated throughout the complement system. Specific activation of the classical pathway is guaranteed by the requirement of specific antibody to bind the foreign antigen. The activation of C1 requires the direct interaction with the antigen-bound antibody (Chapter 2, Section 1). C3 and C4 have a built-in molecular architecture in the form of an extremely reactive thiolester to confer both non-specificity, in its capacity to mediate covalent binding of C3b and C4b to all cell surfaces that carry hydroxyl and amino groups, and specificity, in its rapid inactivation in water so that its only possible covalent binding surface is the same one on which converting enzymes are found (Chapter 2, Section 2). Intrinsic, short-lived convertases, both as C4b,2a and C4b,2a,3b by the dissociation of the C2a component from these complexes, put temporal restriction on complement-mediated activities. Activation of the alternative pathway begins with a low grade non-specific activation of C3 resulting in the random binding of low levels of C3b to all cell surfaces. To ensure that even this minute amount of C3b deposition on host cells does not activate the amplification loop of the alternative pathway, host cells are protected by a range of membrane proteins which interact with C3b and accelerate the dissociation of Bb from potential C3 convertases and also act as cofactors in the permanent inactivation of C3b by factor I (Chapter 2, Section 3). The ability of the terminal complex to disrupt lipid bilayers demonstrates yet another universal mechanism to eliminate membrane-enclosed organisms (Chapter 2, Section 5). The specificity of its activity is again governed by control proteins. The plasma protein, S, which binds and inactivates any fluid phase terminal complex, places a limit to the effective range of the terminal complex from its site of activation (Chapter 2, Section 6.4). Homologous restriction factors, found in most cells, actively protect the cells from damage caused by terminal complexes formed from proteins of the same species (Chapter 2, Section 6.4).

Evolution of such a complex system clearly does not arise from a random process. The coordination can be reflected from the grouping of the complement proteins by their functional and structural properties as discussed in Chapter 3. Furthermore, significant numbers of the 'like' proteins are encoded by linked genes, emphasizing the common origin of these proteins by genomic events like duplication, cross-over and gene conversion. That complement is not an isolated system is reflected in the shared structural and functional features of the complement proteins and those in other systems. The proteases of the complement system may be regarded as regulated and specialized serine proteases (Chapter 3, Section 1). Short consensus repeats (SCRs), though accounting for the entire structural organization of some control proteins in complement such as factor H, are also found in combination with the serine protease domains in C2, factor B, C1r and C1s. It is also found in non-complement proteins such as clotting factor XIII (Chapter 3, Section 4). C3, C4 and C5 are clearly related but differ in that C5 does not have the internal thiolester which accounts for the ability of C3 and C4 to bind covalently to a wide range of cell surfaces. This thiolester is found in a group of related protease inhibitors including α_2-macroglobulin and the pregnancy zone protein (Chapter 3, Section 3). C6, C7, C8 and C9 show sequence homology with each other and perforin (the membranolytic molecule of the cellular immune system). They also contain structural elements similar to those found in low density lipoprotein receptors (Chapter 3, Section 5). The type 3 receptor, CR3, not only shares a subunit with two other cell surface antigens, p150,95 and LFA-1, but also shares structural and functional resemblance to a group of adhesion proteins that bind fibronectin and vitronectin (Chapter 3, Section 6). Finally, the collagen-like part of C1q is responsible for its interaction with the C1q receptor, which possibly has affinity for collagen in general.

Complement does not function as an isolated system either; some of its proteins or the activation products also play essential roles in other physiological reactions. The C1-inhibitor (C1-Inh) regulates plasmin as well as proteases of the clotting system; the anaphylatoxins induce a variety of cellular responses under the description of 'inflammation' (Chapter 4, Section 3); fragments of C3 may serve to regulate the cellular response in the production of antibodies (Chapter 4, Section 7); the binding of C1q to its receptor may inhibit the production of interleukin 1; and CR3 may act as a general receptor on phagocytes, recognizing structures in addition to its complement ligand iC3b (Chapter 3, Section 6).

Research involving the components of the complement system is at an exciting stage given the recent availability of cDNA and genomic clones for most, if not all, the components, control proteins and major receptors associated with the system. Thus, future research will be able to make use of the cloned DNA in a wide variety of studies such as:

(i)   identification of cis-acting, and possibly trans-acting, elements controlling gene expression—as has been initiated by the study of the 5′ flanking regions of the factor B and C2 genes,

(ii)   site-directed mutagenesis studies allowing precise definition of the roles of the small number of residues involved in the formation and control of specificity of the thiolester site in C4,

(iii)   shuffling of whole exons coding for the SCRs found in the C3/C4-binding plasma proteins could provide some insight into the structure – function relationships of the members of the regulators of complement action and expression of altered or truncated versions of cloned receptor molecules should help identify functionally important regions of these molecules,

(iv)   expression of biologically active complement fragments (as has already been achieved for C5a) should provide material completely free of any possible contamination by other complement components/fragments for a variety of studies,

(v)   expression of modified fragments of synthesis of peptides which could be used to control activation, or as inhibitors of inflammation or modulators of the immune response, and

(vi)   availability of the cloned normal gene should help to identify rapidly the precise location of genetic defects in deficiency states.

Studies of this type, making use of the most recent tools of molecular biology, along with physical studies of the enzyme complexes and perhaps crystallization of other complement components or fragments (as has been achieved for the C3a fragment), should allow major advances in the understanding of the complement system in the next few years.

Glossary

Activation of complement: the process by which enzymatically active complement fragments and the membrane attack complex are generated.

Alternative pathway/amplification loop: a pathway which results in C3 activation involving factors B, P, D and C3b, and which is triggered in the presence of activator molecules and surfaces such as components of bacterial and fungal cell walls. In the presence of activators the pathway activation is self-reinforcing and therefore acts to amplify the initial C3 activation, hence it is referred to as an amplification loop.

Anaphylatoxins: the fragments C3a and C5a which, by their actions on the vasculature and smooth muscle, produce symptoms of anaphylaxis.

Chemotaxis: the directional movement of cells up a concentration gradient of a chemotactic molecule.

Classical pathway: a pathway which results in C3 activation, involving C1, C2 and C4, which is triggered by antigen – antibody complexes, binding to C1q.

Complement receptors: cellular receptors for various fragments of complement molecules generated during activation.

Convertases: molecular complexes which can enzymatically cleave particular components (e.g. C3 convertases split C3 into C3a and C3b).

Enzyme cascade: a description of several plasma enzyme systems, including complement, in which the activation of one component generates an enzyme which acts on the next component in the activation sequence.

Kinins: a group of molecules which act on blood vessels causing increased vascular permeability and increased blood flow.

Membrane attack complex (MAC): a molecular complex formed by C5b, C6, C7, C8 and a number of C9 molecules which can integrate into plasma membranes and may cause cell lysis.

MHC class III genes: a region of the major histocompatibility complex which encodes genes not involved in T cell immune recognition (i.e. not class I and II genes). This includes the genes for C4, C2, factor B and 21-hydroxylase.

Opsonization: the process by which antigenic material becomes coated with molecules (e.g. C3b) which facilitate uptake by phagocytes.

Perforins: proteins which are secreted by cytotoxic T cells and which are involved in causing lysis of target cells.

Pro-enzyme: an enzymatically inactive molecule which may become enzymatically active following intracellular processing or internal cleavage.

Restriction fragment length polymorphism (RFLP): genetic variation between individuals, analysed by nicking the DNA at specific sites with restriction enzymes and analysing the lengths of the fragments produced.

Terminal pathway (lytic pathway): the pathway involving C5 – C9 which generates the membrane attack complex.

Thiolester: the chemical structure $-S-CO-$. In the case of the complement proteins C3 and C4, the bond is formed between a $-SH$ group on a cysteine residue and a $-CONH_2$ group on a glutamine residue with the elimination of NH_3.

Index